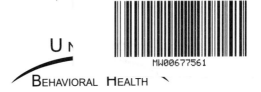

To: UBH Network Clinicians

From: Saul Feldman, CEO
Carol Shaw, VP Provider Services

Re: Clinical Evidence

Date: February 2001

The amount of information on behavioral health care that is available today through the professional and popular media is overwhelming and much of it can be fragmentary and confusing. This makes it difficult for clinicians to discern which information is based on sound and current scientific evidence and which is not.

We want to help you obtain evidence-based information that can be used to improve patient care. As part of this effort, we are pleased to provide you with the mental health supplement of *Clinical Evidence*, an international resource that provides easy access to the most up-to-date information on what works in health care. It was developed by the BMJ Publishing Group, publisher of the 160-year old *British Medical Journal*, in conjunction with internationally recognized experts.

Clinical Evidence does not tell you what to do. Rather, it provides the best evidence to help clinicians and patients decide on the most appropriate course of action. The unique format is designed to allow you to interpret the evidence and make the appropriate decision based on a particular situation.

The BMJ Publishing Group is solely responsible for the content of all issues of *Clinical Evidence* and is continually revising it based on feedback from clinicians. I encourage you to provide them with comments via CEfeedback@bmjgroup.com.

I hope that this supplement of *Clinical Evidence* is helpful to you. Please feel free to let me know what you think of it.

FEBRUARY 2001

clinical evidence Mental Health

The international source of the best available evidence in mental health care

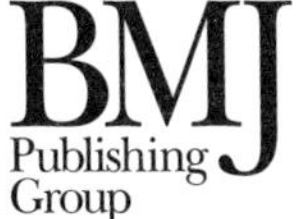

Clinical Evidence *Mental Health*

Editorial Office
BMJ Publishing Group, BMA House, Tavistock Square, London, WC1H 9JR, United Kingdo
Tel: +44 (0)20 7387 4499 Fax: +44 (0)20 7383 6242 www.bmjpg.com

Subscription rates
The complete edition of *Clinical Evidence* is published on a six monthly basis (June/December). The annual subscription rates for Issues 4 & 5 (December 2000 and June 2001) are:

Individual: US$110 / Can$160
Institutional: US$240 / Can$345
Student: US$80 / Can $120

The above rates include print and online formats for individuals and students. The institutional rate is for print only. Institutions may purchase online site licenses separately. For further information visit the subscription pages of our website www.clinicalevidence.org or contact Diane McCabe, US Product Manager dmccabe@bmjgroup.com

All subscriptions to BMJ-Clinical Evidence, PO Box 512, Annapolis Jct, MD 20701-0512, USA. Tel: 1-800-373-2897/1-240-646-7000 • Fax: 1-240-646-7005 • Email: clinevid@pmds.com
Alternatively, you can visit the BMJ Publishing Group website to order online www.bmjpg.com

Bulk subscriptions for societies and organisations
The Publishers offer discounts for any society or organisation buying bulk quantities for the members/specific groups. Please contact Diane McCabe at dmccabe@bmjgroup.com

Feedback
We are always looking to improve *Clinical Evidence* to make it as useful, accurate, and up to date as possible. Please give us your views, comments, and suggestions. You can email us at CEfeedback@bmjgroup.com

Contributors
If you are interested in becoming a contributor to *Clinical Evidence* please contact us at clinicalevidence@bmjgroup.com

Clinical Evidence Online
Clinical Evidence is available online. Register now at ww.clinicalevidence.org for free access. For information about electronic products, including access through Ovid and a standalone intranet version, please contact Rachel Armitage at clinicalevidence@bmjgroup.com

Rights
For information on translation rights, please contact Daniel Raymond-Barker at clinicalevidence@bmjgroup.com

Permission to reproduce
Please email Josephine Woodcock at clinicalevidence@bmjgroup.com to request permission to reprint all or part of any contribution in *Clinical Evidence*.

Legal Disclaimer
Care has been taken to confirm the accuracy of the information presented and to describe generally accepted practices. However, the authors, editors, and publishers are not responsible for errors or omissions or for any consequences from application of the information in this book and make no warranty, express or implied, with respect to the contents of the publication.

Printed by The Sheridan Press, Hanover, Pennsylvania, USA.

;linical Evidence team and advisors

;ontents

About Clinical Evidence

Clinical Evidence is a regularly updated compendium of evidence on the effects of clinical interventions. It summarises the current state of knowledge, ignorance, and uncertainty about the prevention and treatment of clinical conditions, based on thorough searches and appraisal of the literature. It is not a text book of medicine nor a book of guidelines. It describes the best available evidence, and where there is no good evidence, it says so. *Clinical Evidence* is curently updated every six months, and expanded to include summaries of the evidence on additional diseases, syndromes, and clinical questions.

Clinical Evidence has several unique features:

- Its contents are driven by questions rather than by the availability of research evidence. Rather than start with the evidence and summarise what is there, important clinical questions are identified and the literature searched for the best availble evidence to answer them.
- It identifies but does not try to fill important gaps in the evidence.
- It is updated every six months. This means that you can rely on it to keep you up to date in the areas that are covered.
- It specifically aims not to make recommendations because differences in individual patients' baseline risks and preferences, and in the local availability of interventions, will always mean that the evidence must be individually interpreted rather than applied across the board.

Clinical Evidence works alongside *Evidence Based Mental Health* (http://www.ebmentalhealth.com)[1] to provide the best, up-to-date evidence for clinicians. We hope you find it useful as an aid to clinical decision making and welcome your feedback.

Welcome to Clinical Evidence Mental Health

Welcome to the Mental Health version of *Clinical Evidence*. This section is reprinted from *Clinical Evidence* and is meant for psychiatrists, psychologists, nurses, social workers, and therapists working in a mental health setting.

Mental health has long been a field led by passionate opinions. An evidence-based approach in mental health is perhaps more challenging than other medical disciplines because of the very nature of the profession and interventions used. Narrative-based approaches are an important part of the therapeutic interaction between patient and therapist,[2] and the patient's story and environment can best be appreciated with a narrative approach.[3]

The challenge to mental health professionals is to synthesise the clinical experience with the "concientious, explicit and judicious use of evidence to make treatment decisions",[4] including the patients and, where appropriate, their families or carers in the process. The discussion of evidence with patients should occur whenever a clinical decision affecting the care of an individual patient is considered. That is the basis of informed consent and, indeed, of clinical care. Evidence-based mental health is not "cook-book" or "cost cutting medicine". Evidence will emphasise systematic reviews and randomised controlled trials (RCTs) for many situations, but is not restricted to these as the appropriate method depends on the clinical question being answered.[4]

The application of evidence in mental health includes the following barriers: (1) the task of monitoring the literature ('data smog'), with over 40 000 biomedical journals and that amount doubling every 20 years;[5] (2) the practicalities of implementation of research into practice;[6] (3) the poor acceptance of RCTs in psychiatry;[7] (4) the paucity of evidence-based treatment guidelines; (5) the conflicting interpretations of evidence within mental health,[7,8] leaving clinicians "on a tightrope act between the persuasiveness of the marketing claims, the precise but somewhat myopic results of idealised clinical trials, and the complex realities of clinical practice";[9–11] (6) the difficulty in standardising outcomes in RCTs in mental health;[7] and (7) the challenge of study design, particularly for psychological treatments where RCTs are often small, of short duration, and susceptible to bias.[7] Furthermore, the field of mental health and particularly the treatments used may often be subject to the effects of media and popular opinion,[11] to bias within the profession,[13] to publication bias, and to the influence of pharmaceutical companies.[13] Thornley and Adams[15] reviewed the quality of 2000 published RCTs in schizophrenia and found most to be dominated by underpowered pharmacological studies often commercially sponsored. The interpretation of individual RCTs may also be subject to bias.[16] The production of systematic reviews[17] and the textual interpretation[18] may further decorate by the authors' values in all fields of mental health.

However, one has only to be briefly reminded of the history of non-evidence-based treatments in mental health to appreciate the need for use of evidence in decision making in treating mental illness. They include the injudicious use of restraints, psychosurgery, malaria therapy (for which Julius Wagner-Jauregg won a Noble Prize — the only psychiatrist to ever do so!), insulin coma therapy, and ECT for clinical conditions for which it has not been shown to have effect. All of these have greatly contributed to the stigma of both psychiatric patients and psychiatrists, and have held back progress in mental health well behind that of other medical disciplines.[19] Evidence must be incorporated into daily practice in order to avoid repeating history. The use of evidence in mental health can help to provide better patient care and to shape what research is needed to make rational clinical decisions.

Evidence-based medicine and mental health is slowly being incorporated into daily clinical decisions. Field and Lohe[20] estimate that a total of 45% of clinical decisions would be based on very weak or no evidence, 25% on modest evidence and consensus, and 20% on modest evidence but strong consensus, with only 4% of decisions which might be made on the basis of strong evidence and 6% on the basis of very weak or no evidence or consensus at all. One study has estimated that 65% of decisions in an acute adult inpatient psychiatric setting were based on RCT evidence[21] and another found 53% of treatment decisions based on RCT evidence,[22] both using retrospective searches of the literature. Booth points to estimates ranging from 10% to 70% of medicine having an RCT evidence base.[23] This does not reflect the numbers of psychiatrists practising evidence-based medicine — rather only the percentage of clinical decisions for which evidence could be found to back up the clinical decision! While the uptake in daily practice is growing slowly, the use of 'evidence-based purchasing' in mental health is likely to increase rapidly[24] as cost effectiveness takes on greater importance. One must hope that administrators and managers will not jump to the conclusion that a scarcity of evidence necessarily implies lack of efficacy.[16] We have made every effort to emphasise the reporting of effects — i.e. balancing the evidence of benefits and harms — and not merely effectiveness in *Clinical Evidence*.

The chapters here are the result of a rigorous process aimed at ensuring that the information they contain is both reliable and relevant to clinical practice. We have specifically chosen questions in mental health that put the emphasis on outcomes that matter to patients and clinicians. We therefore use specific clinical measures as outcomes whenever possible such as symptom severity, quality of life, survival, and disability, and avoid using trials using proxy or non-clinical outcomes such as laboratory values.

Putting the evidence together

The literature is searched using the Cochrane Library, Medline, Embase, Psychlit and, occasionally, other electronic databases, looking first for good systematic reviews of RCTs then for good RCTs published since the search date of the review. Where we find no good recent systematic review, we search for all individual RCTs. The studies that are identified in the search are critically appraised by two information scientists working independently and using validated criteria similar to those of Sackett et al[25] and Jadad.[26,27] Where the search identifies more than one or two good systematic reviews or trials, we select those we judge to be the most robust or relevant, using the full text of the article. Where we identify few or no good reviews or trials, we include other studies but highlight their limitations.

Contributors are experts in both the clinical field being reviewed and in epidemiology. They start by setting the questions that clinicians need to know in the clinical situation. They then review our selection of studies, and are asked to justify any additions or exclusions they wish to make. All competing interests are made explicit in each chapter. Based on the search, the contributors then summarise the evidence relating to each question. Each topic is then peer reviewed by the section advisors, by at least three external expert clinicians and discussed at length at a teleconferenced editorial meeting. Finally, the revised text is reviewed by editors with clinical and epidemiological training, and data are checked against the original study reports whenever necessary. Whenever possible, data are presented in the same form as in the original studies. However, sometimes we have changed the units or type of information used to allow comparison with results from other studies and will, for example, convert odds ratios into relative risks where appropriate.

The summaries for each chapter include a categorisation of the treatment options that we have modified from one of the Cochrane Collaboration's first and most popular products, *A guide to effective care in pregnancy and childbirth*.[27] These categories are explained in the table below:

TABLE Categorisation of treatment effects in *Clinical Evidence*

Beneficial	Interventions whose effectiveness has been demonstrated by clear evidence from randomised controlled trials, and expectation of harms that is small compared with the benefits.
Likely to be beneficial	Interventions for which effectiveness is less well established than for those listed under "beneficial".
Trade off between benefits and harms	Interventions for which clinicians and patients should weigh up the beneficial and harmful effects according to individual circumstances and priorities.
Unknown effectiveness	Interventions for which there are currently insufficient data or data of inadequate quality (includes interventions that are widely accepted as beneficial but have never been formally tested in RCTs, often because RCTs would be considered unethical).
Unlikely to be beneficial	Interventions for which lack of effectiveness is less well established than for those listed under "likely to be ineffective or harmful".
Likely to be ineffective or harmful	Interventions whose ineffectiveness or harmfulness has been demonstrated by clear evidence.

Categorising interventions takes into account not only the level of evidence of benefit, but also the potential harms and degree of certainty around the finding (represented by the confidence interval). Much of the evidence that is most relevant to clinical decisions relates to comparisons between different interventions rather than to comparison with placebo or no intervention or to specific populations, and the specific treatment comparisons are indicated where appropriate.

As many of the treatments available in the field of mental health have not been subjected to good RCTs, we will frequently report finding limited or no evidence for many options. Saying that there is no good evidence that a treatment works is not the same as saying that the treatment doesn't work. It should be emphasised that these statements are a reflection of the published literature available at the time of the search and not a statement about whether or not an intervention is effective. We have thus made every effort in the text to distinguish between a lack of benefit and a lack of evidence of benefit.

A key aim of *Clinical Evidence* is to emphasise the important trade offs between the benefits and harms of different interventions. We therefore talk about the effects of interventions, both positive and negative, rather than the effectiveness; and for each intervention we present evidence on 'benefits' and 'harms'. 'Harms' include adverse effects of treatment and inconvenience to the patient.

We make no attempt to provide information on drug dosages, formulations, indications, and contraindications. For this information, we refer readers to their national drug formularies. Drug dosages are included only when a question explores the relative effects of different doses. We have decided not to include information on the cost or cost effectiveness of interventions because costs vary greatly both within and between countries.

We hope you find *Clinical Evidence* Mental Health a useful aid to clinical decision making and welcome your feedback.

Harry McConnell MD FRCPC
Clinical Editor, Mental Health Section

REFERENCES

1. Geddes J, Reynolds S, Streiner D, Szatmari P. Evidence based practice in mental health. *BMJ* 1997;315.
2. Launer J. A narrative approach to mental health in general practice. *BMJ* 1999;318:117–119.
3. Holmes J. Can narrative approaches help in our understanding and management of psychosis? *Acta Psychiatr Scand* 2000;102:1.
4. Sackett DL, Rosenberg WMC, Gray JAM, Haynes RB, Richardson WS. Evidence-Based Medicine: What it is and what it isn't. *BMJ* 1996;312:71–72.
5. Wyatt J. Reading journals and monitoring the published work. *J R Soc Med* 2000;93:423–427.
6. Sheldon TA, Gilbody SM. Invited commentaries on closing the gap between research and practice. *Br J Psychiatry* 1997;171:226–227.
7. Andrews A. Randomised controlled trials in psychiatry: important but poorly accepted. *BMJ* 1999;319:562–564.
8. Barker H. Trials show that psychotherapy is effective for wide range of psychological conditions. *BMJ* 2000;320:186.
9. Kapur S, Remington G. Atypical antipsychotics. *BMJ* 2000;321:1360–1361.
10. Geddes J, Freemantle N, Harrison P, Bebbington P. Atypical antipsychotics in the treatment of schizophrenia: a systematic overview and meta-regression analysis. *BMJ* 2000;321:1371–1376.
11. Adams C. Typical vs atypicals: bad science in the BMJ. http://www.bmj.com; 8 Dec 2000 [Response].
12. Ciment J. Consumer group criticises surgeon. *BMJ* 1999;319:1092.
13. Anderson I. Psychiatry: evidence-based but still value-laden. *Br J Psychiatry* 1997;171:226–227.
14. Gilbody SM, Song F. Publication bias and the integrity of psychiatry research. *Psychol Med* 2000;30:253–258.
15. Thornley B, Adams C. Content and quality of 2000 controlled trials in schizophrenia over 50 years. *BMJ* 1998;317: 1181–1184.
16. Milton J, Richardson P, Hale R. Scarcity of evidence is not necessarily evidence against long term psychodynamic psychotherapy. *BMJ* 2000;320:186.
17. Sikdar S. Evidence-based psychiatry: which evidence to believe? *Br J Psychiatry* 1997;171:483–484.
18. Horton R. The rhetoric of research. *BMJ* 1995;310:985–987.
19. Valenstein, Elliot, Great and Desparate Cures: *The rise and decline of psychosurgery and other radical treatments for mental illness*. New York: Basic Books, 1986.
20. Field MJ, Lohe KN, eds. *Guidelines for clinical practice: from development to use by committee on clinical practice guidelines*. Washington: National Academy of Science, Institute of Medicine, 1992.

21. Geddes JR, Game D, Jenkins NE, Peterson LA, Pottinger GR, Sackett DL. What proportion of primary psychiatric interventions are based on evidence from randomised controlled trials? *Qual Health Care* 1996; 4:215–217.
22. Summers A, Kehoe RF. Is psychiatric treatment evidence-based [letter]? *Lancet* 1996; 347:409–410.
23. Booth A. What proportion of healthcare is evidence based? Resource guide. http://www.shef.ac.uk/~scharr/ir/percent.html [accessed 12 January 2001].
24. Kisley S. Psychotherapy for severe personality disorder: exploring the limits of evidence based purchasing. *BMJ* 1999; 318:1410–1412.
25. Sackett DL, Haynes RB, Guyatt GH, Tugwell P. *Clinical Epidemiology: A basic science for clinical medicine*. 2nd ed. Boston: Little Brown, 1991.
26. Jadad A. Assessing the quality of RCTs: Why, what, how and by whom? In: Jadad A. *Randomised Controlled Trials*. London: BMJ Books, 1998:45–60.
27. Jadad AR, Moore RA, Carroll D, Jenkinson C, et al. Assessing the quality of reports of randomized clinical trials: is blinding necessary? *Control Clin Trials* 1996;17:1–12.
28. Enkin M, Keirse M, Renfrew M, et al. *A guide to effective care in pregnancy and childbirth*. Oxford: Oxford University Press, 1998.

Clinical Evidence Glossary

Absolute risk (AR) This is the probability that an individual will experience the specified outcome during a specified period. It lies in the range 0 to 1. In contrast to common usage, the word 'risk' may refer to adverse events (such as myocardial infarction), or desirable events (such as cure).
Absolute risk reduction (ARR) The absolute difference in risk between the experimental and control groups in a trial, where risk in the control group is higher. Absolute risk increase (ARI) The absolute difference in risk between the experimental and control groups in a trial, where risk in the experimental group is higher.
Bias Systematic deviation of study results from the true results, due to the way(s) in which the study is conducted.
Case control study A study design that examines a group of people who have experienced an event (usually an adverse event) and a group of people who have not experienced the same event, and looks at how exposure to suspect (usually noxious) agents differed between the two groups.
Clinically significant A finding that is clinically important. Here, 'significant' takes its everyday meaning of 'important' (compare with statistically significant, see below). Where the word 'significant' or 'significance' is used without qualification in the text, it is being used in its statistical sense.
Cohort study A non-experimental study design that follows a group of people (a cohort), and then looks at how events differ among people within the group. A study that examines two cohorts, one that has been exposed to a suspect agent or treatment, and one that has not been exposed, is useful for trying to ascertain whether exposure is likely to cause specified events (often adverse). Prospective cohort studies (which track participants forward in time) are more reliable than retrospective cohort studies (which look back in time to ascertain whether or not participants were exposed to the agent in question).
Completer analysis Analysis of data from only those participants who remained at the end of the study. Compare with intention to treat analysis, which uses data from all participants who enrolled (see below).
Confidence interval (CI) The 95% confidence interval (or 95% confidence limits) would include 95% of results from studies of the same size and design. This is close but not identical to saying that the true size of the effect (never exactly known) has a 95% chance of falling within the confidence interval. If the 95% CI for a relative risk or an odds ratio crosses 1, the effect size is likely to lie in a range where risk is either increased or decreased.
Controls in a randomised controlled trial refer to the participants in its comparison group. They are allocated either to placebo, to no treatment, or to the standard treatment.
Cross sectional study A study design that involves surveying a population about an exposure, or condition, or both, at one point in time. It can be used for assessing prevalence of a condition in the population.
Effect size Many methods are used to quantify the size of an effect. For dichotomous outcomes, relative risk and odds ratio are examples. Typically, the term effect size is used for continuous variables (such as pain scores or height), where the standardised mean difference or weighted mean difference (see below) are commonly used.
Event The occurrence of a dichotomous outcome that is being sought in the study (such as myocardial infarction, death, or a four-point improvement in pain score).
Hazard ratio (HR) This is broadly equivalent to relative risk, but is used when the risk is not constant with respect to time.
Heterogeneity In the context of meta-analysis, heterogeneity means dissimilarity between studies. It can be due to use of different statistical methods (statistical heterogeneity), or evaluation of different types of patients, treatments or outcomes (clinical heterogeneity). Heterogeneity may render pooling of data in meta-analysis unreliable or inappropriate.
Homogeneity Similarity (see heterogeneity).

Incidence The number of new cases of a condition occurring in a population over a specified period of time.

Intention to treat analysis Analysis of data from all participants who were enrolled into the study as if they had remained in the group into which they were randomised, regardless of whether they actually remained until the end or withdrew from the trial. Compare with completer analysis (see above).

Meta-analysis A statistical technique that summarises the results of several studies in a single weighted estimate, in which more weight is given to results from larger studies.

Morbidity Rate of illness but not death.

Mortality Rate of death.

Number needed to treat (NNT) One measure of treatment effectiveness. It is the number of people you would need to treat with a specific intervention for a given period of time to prevent one additional adverse outcome or achieve one additional beneficial outcome. NNT can be calculated as 1/ARR (see appendix 2).

Number needed to harm (NNH) One measure of treatment harm. It is the number of people you would need to treat with a specific intervention for a given period of time to cause one additional adverse outcome. NNH can be calculated as 1/ARI.

Odds ratio (OR) One measure of treatment effectiveness. It is the odds of an event happening in the experimental group, expressed as a proportion of the odds of an event happening in the control group. The closer the OR is to one, the smaller the difference in effect between the experimental intervention and the control intervention. If the OR is greater (or less) than one, then the effects of the treatment are more (or less) than those of the control treatment. Note that the effects being measured may be adverse (e.g. death or disability) or desirable (e.g. survival). When events are rare, the OR is analagous to the relative risk (RR), but as event rates increase, the OR and RR diverge.

Odds reduction The complement of odds ratio (1-OR), similar to the relative risk reduction (RRR) when events are rare.

P value The probability that an observed difference occurred by chance, if it is assumed that there is in fact no underlying difference between the means of the observations. If this probability is less than 1 in 20 (which is when the P value is less than 0.05), then the result is conventionally regarded as being "statistically significant".

Placebo A substance given in the control group of a clinical trial ideally identical in appearance and taste or feel to the experimental treatment and without any disease specific effects. The term is sometimes applied in the context of non-pharmacological interventions.

Prevalence The proportion of people with a finding or disease in a given population at a given time.

Publication bias occurs when studies with positive results being more likely to be published than studies with negative results, so making it appear from surveys of the published literature that treatments are more effective than is truly the case.

Randomised controlled trial (RCT) A trial in which participants are randomly assigned to two groups: one (the experimental group) receiving the intervention that is being tested, and the other (the comparison or control group) receiving an alternative treatment or placebo. This design allows assessment of the relative effects of interventions.

Relative risk (RR) The number of times more likely (RR greater than 1) or less likely (RR less than 1) an event is likely to happen in one group compared with another. It is analogous to the odds ratio (OR) when events are rare, and is the ratio of the absolute risk for each group. **Relative risk increase (RRI)** The proportional increase in risk between experimental and control participants in a trial. **Relative risk reduction (RRR)** The proportional reduction in risk between experimental and control participants in a trial. It is the complement of the relative risk (1-RR).

Significant By convention taken to mean statistically significant at the 5% level (see statistically significant).

Standardised mean difference (SMD) A measure of effect size used when outcomes are continuous (such as height, weight, or symptom scores) rather than dichotomous (such as death or myocardial infarction). The mean differences in outcome between the groups being studied are standardised to account for differences in scoring methods (such as pain scores). The measure is a ratio, and therefore has no units.

Statistically significant means that the findings of a study are unlikely to be due to chance. Significance at the commonly cited 5% level ($P < 0.05$) means that the observed result would occur by chance in only 1 in 20 similar studies. Where the word "significant" or "significance" is used without qualification in the text, it is being used in this statistical sense.

Systematic review A review in which the trials on a topic have been systematically identified, appraised, and summarised according to predetermined criteria. It can, but need not, involve meta-analysis as a statistical method of adding together and numerically summarising the results of the trials that meet minimum quality criteria.

Validity The soundness or rigour of a study. Internal Validity refers to the way a study is designed and carried out. It means that the results are unbiased and give you an accurate estimate of the effect that is being measured. External Validity refers to the aqpplication of the results of a trial outside it's original context.

Weighted mean difference (WMD) A measure of effect size used when outcomes are continuous (such as symptom scores or height) rather than dichotomous (such as death or myocardial infarction). The mean differences in outcome between the groups being studied are weighted to account for different sample sizes and differing precision between studies. The WMD is an absolute figure, and so takes the units of the original outcome measure.

Alzheimer's disease

James Warner and Rob Butler

QUESTIONS

INTERVENTIONS

To be covered in future issues of *Clinical Evidence*
Aspirin
Oestrogen
Risperidone
Vitamin E
Music therapy
Treatment of other types of dementia

See glossary, p 7

Key Messages

- Most RCTs used proxy outcome measures such as cognitive function, rather than clinical outcomes likely to be important to people with Alzheimer's disease and their carers, such as quality of life.
- Systematic reviews of RCTs have found:
  - Improved cognitive function and global clinical state with donepezil 10 mg compared with placebo. Treatment is well tolerated.
  - Improved cognitive function with rivastigmine 6–12 mg; possibly less effective than donepezil. Nausea is common.
  - No evidence that tacrine improves cognitive function or behaviour. In trials, tacrine is associated with hepatotoxicity.
  - Reduced anxiety with short term treatment with thioridazine, but no evidence of an effect on clinical global state. A link between thioridazine and cardiac arrhythmias has been suggested.
  - Improved cognitive function, behaviour, and mood with selegiline compared with placebo, but no evidence of an effect on clinical global state; treatment is well tolerated with no serious adverse events.
  - Improved cognitive function with ginkgo biloba. Treatment is well tolerated.
- One small RCT found no benefit from diclofenac compared with placebo.
- One systematic review of small RCTs found that reality orientation is associated with improved cognitive function and behaviour compared with no treatment.
- We found insufficient evidence on the effects of reminisence therapy.

Alzheimer's disease

DEFINITION **Dementia** is characterised by global impairment of cerebral function with preservation of clear consciousness. It usually results in loss of memory (initially of recent events), loss of executive function (such as the ability to make decisions or sequence complex tasks), and changes in personality. **Alzheimer's disease** is characterised by an insidious onset and slow deterioration, and may be diagnosed after other systemic and neurological causes of dementia have been excluded clinically and by laboratory investigation.

INCIDENCE/ PREVALENCE About 5% of people aged over 65 years and 20% of people aged over 80 years have some form of dementia.[1] Dementia is rare before the age of 60. The most common type of dementia is Alzheimer's disease, accounting for about 60% of cases in the UK.[2] The rest comprise mainly vascular dementia, mixed vascular and Alzheimer's disease, and cortical Lewy body dementia.[3]

AETIOLOGY/ RISK FACTORS The cause of Alzheimer's disease is poorly understood. A key pathological process is thought to be a defect in amyloid precursor protein leading to deposition of abnormal amyloid in the central nervous system.[4] Most cases of the relatively rare condition of early onset dementia (before age 60) show autosomal dominance. Later onset dementia sometimes clusters in families. Vascular dementia is related to cardiovascular risk factors, such as smoking, hypertension, and diabetes.

PROGNOSIS Alzheimer's disease usually has an insidious onset when it is often difficult to diagnose. There is inexorable reduction in cerebral function over time, with an average life expectancy after diagnosis of 7–10 years.[3] Behavioural problems, depression, and psychosis occur in most people at some stage.[5,6] Eventually, most people with dementia find it difficult to perform simple tasks without help.

AIMS To improve cognitive function (memory, orientation, attention, and concentration); to reduce behavioural problems (wandering and aggression); to improve quality of life, with minimum adverse effects of treatment.

OUTCOMES Quality of life both of the person with dementia and their carer (rarely used in clinical trials). Comprehensive scales of cognitive function such as the Alzheimer's disease assessment scale cognitive subscale (ADAS-cog, where lower scores signify improving function)[7] are more sensitive than briefer scales such as the mini-mental status examination (MMSE),[8] but both are proxy measures that may not reflect outcomes important to people with dementia or their careers. A seven point change in the ADAS-cog may be regarded as clinically significant. Overall condition is reflected in scales such as global clinical state. One measure of global state is the clinician interview-based impression of change with caregiver input (CIBIC-Plus) scale. Psychiatric symptoms are assessed using scales such as the dementia mood assessment scale (DMAS) and the brief psychiatric rating scale (BPRS) (both of which use lower scores to signify improved symptoms). Other outcomes include time to institutionalisation or death.

METHODS *Clinical Evidence* update search and appraisal May 2000. All relevant systematic reviews and RCTs were reviewed.

QUESTION What are the effects of drug treatments?

OPTION CHOLINESTERASE INHIBITORS

One systematic review of RCTs has found evidence that donepezil is well tolerated and is better than placebo in improving cognitive function and global clinical state. One systematic review of RCTs has found no evidence of benefit from tacrine in terms of improved cognitive function or behaviour. Tacrine has also been associated with hepatotoxicity. One large RCT found that rivastigmine is associated with improved cognitive function in older people with Alzheimer's disease but that nausea was common. We found no evidence that any of the drugs significantly improved quality of life.

Benefits: **Donepezil:** We found one systematic review (search date 2000), which identified three placebo controlled RCTs evaluating cholinesterase inhibitors.[9] The trials included 1102 people with mild or moderate Alzheimer's disease. The review found that donepezil 10 mg was associated with improved cognitive function, measured by the ADAS-cog score (WMD –3.01, 95% CI –3.92 to –2.09; 5 mg: WMD –2.61, 95% CI –3.45 to –1.78) and improved global clinical state (OR 0.38, 95% CI 0.26 to 0.56). There was no evidence of an effect on self rated quality of life. One 24 week double blind RCT included in the systematic review, comparing 10 mg donezepil with placebo in 473 people with mild to moderate Alzheimer's disease, found that the NNT was 4 for a four point improvement in ADAS-cog and 6 for a seven point improvement.[10] We found one subsequent 30 week RCT (818 people with Alzheimer's) comparing donepezil 10 mg versus donepezil 5 mg versus placebo. It found improved global state to be associated with both donepezil treatments (NNT 10, 95% CI 6 to 25 with donepezil 10 mg *v* placebo for a three point improvement in CIBIC score). It found no evidence of a difference in quality of life.[11] **Tacrine:** We found one systematic review (search date November 1998), which identified five placebo controlled RCTs in 1434 people.[12] Various dosages of tacrine were given for 1–39 weeks. The review found no significant difference in overall clinical improvement (OR 0.87, 95% CI 0.61 to 1.23), a significant (but probably clinically insignificant) improvement in cognition (WMD in ADAS-cog –0.22, 95% CI –0.32 to –0.12), and no significant difference in MMSE (SMD 0.14, 95% CI –0.02 to +0.3). There was no evidence of improved behaviour (SMD in behavioural disturbance on the non-cognitive subscale of ADAS –0.04, 95% CI –0.52 to +0.43). **Rivastigmine:** We found one systematic review, which identified seven RCTs (search date 1999).[13] Two of the trials, accounting for 1379 people (49% of all trial people for this drug), remain unpublished and the data were not made available to the reviewers. The review found an NNT of 20 (95 % CI 13 to 50) for a four point change in the ADAS-cog for 6–12 mg rivastigmine compared with placebo. There was no significant difference between 1–4 mg rivastigmine and placebo. One multicentre, placebo controlled RCT evaluated rivastigmine 6–12 mg for 24 weeks in 725 people with probable Alzheimer's disease.[14] It found that significantly more people had a four point improvement in the ADAS-cog score with rivastigmine than with placebo (57/242 [24%] *v* 39/238

[16%] NNT 13 95% CI 7 to 113). The trial found no significant difference between low dose rivastigmine 1–4 mg and placebo for these outcomes.

Harms: **Donepezil** was well tolerated in the trials. The main adverse effects reported were mild and transient nausea, vomiting, and diarrhoea. No hepatotoxicity was reported. More people withdrew from the donepezil 10 mg group than the placebo group (69/315 *v* 43/315, OR 1.79, 95% CI 1.19 to 2.70), although withdrawal rates for donepezil 5 mg versus placebo were similar (12.6% *v* 14.9%).[9] **Tacrine:** Withdrawals were common and related to dosage. Inconsistencies in reporting make it hard to give an overall withdrawal figure. Two studies where this was possible (812 people) gave an odds ratio for withdrawal of 5.7 (95% CI 4.1 to 7.9). In one high dose study, 72% of people taking tacrine 160 mg withdrew.[15] Reversible hepatotoxicity was reported in about half of participants. Diarrhoea, anorexia, and abdominal pain were also common. **Rivastigmine:** One trial reported no serious adverse effects.[14] However, 33% of people taking the high dose withdrew. The most commonly reported adverse effects were nausea (50%), vomiting (34%), dizziness (20%), headache (19%), and diarrhoea (17%).[12]

Comment: The trials all used proxy outcomes (cognitive scores) rather than outcomes likely to be important to people with Alzheimer's disease and their carers. All trials of donepezil used reliable methods, but participants were highly selected and may not be representative. Quality of life of carers was not assessed.[9] The quality of tacrine trials was generally poor. The longest RCT lasted 30 weeks[15] and doses varied considerably between trials. Although the NNT was higher than that for donepezil, rivastigmine is the only cholinesterase inhibitor we found to have been studied in a routine clinical (pragmatic) setting.[14] Data on 49% of all people in the phase II/III trials of rivastigmine have not been reported. As a consequence there may have been an overestimation of the reported treatment effect in the meta-analysis. A significant issue with dementia trials is the way missing data are managed. Many trials show much higher dropout rates (30% or more) at doses where the drug is effective than in the placebo arm. Missing data are often managed using last observation carried forward (LOCF) in these studies. In dementing people, the likely trend over the course of the trial will be to get worse. If people drop out of the trial, relatively better scores are carried forward to end point than if the person completed. If more people drop out of the intervention arm, an artificially better score, compared with the placebo arm, will result.

OPTION THIORIDAZINE

One systematic review of RCTs has found that short term treatment with thioridazine reduces anxiety but found no evidence of an effect on clinical global state. We found only limited data on adverse effects.

Benefits: We found one systematic review (updated 1998, 7 RCTs). Six trials were of 3–4 weeks' duration and one lasted 8 weeks; of the seven, two were placebo controlled.[16] The review found evidence that thioridazine reduced symptoms of anxiety (*v* placebo OR 4.91, 95%

CI 3.12 to 7.50; *v* diazepam OR 1.8, 95% CI 1.04 to 3.10) but did not significantly affect clinical global state (*v* placebo OR 1.58, 95% CI 0.42 to 5.96).

Harms: The trials included in the review did not report adverse events systematically.[16] Adverse effects were no more common with thioridazine than with placebo (OR 0.41, 95% CI 0.09 to 1.86) or diazepam (OR 0.84, 95% CI 0.25 to 2.82). One trial included in the review (60 people) found that people taking thioridazine were less alert than people taking chlormethiazole (OR for alertness 0.31, 95% CI 0.11 to 0.89) and less likely to be continent of urine (OR 0.24, 95% CI 0.07 to 0.69). A link between thioridazine and cardiac arrhythmias has been suggested.[17]

Comment: The dose of thioridazine varied from 10–200 mg. Doses of comparator drugs also varied. The review identified 51 studies.[16] However, all but seven were excluded because of poor quality methods or lack of usable data. All trials were of short duration.

OPTION SELEGILINE

One systematic review of RCTs has found that selegiline is better than placebo at improving cognitive function, behavioural disturbance, and mood in people with Alzheimer's disease. It found no evidence of an effect on clinical global state. Selegiline was well tolerated with no serious adverse events.

Benefits: We found one systematic review (search date 2000), which identified 15 RCTs comparing selegiline versus placebo (average n = 50, typical duration of treatment 3 months).[18] Analysis of pooled data found that selegiline improved several outcome measures: cognitive function scores (as measured by several parameters, SMD –0.56, 95% CI –0.88 to –0.24); mood score (DMAS), SMD –1.14, 95% CI –2.11 to –0.18); and behavioural symptom score (BPRS, SMD –0.53, 95% CI –0.94 to –0.12). However, the review found no evidence of an effect on global rating scales (SMD –0.11, 95% CI –0.49 to +0.27).

Harms: Withdrawal rates were low and, except in one study, no significant difference was found between groups.[19] The trials reported no major adverse events.

Comment: The trials all used proxy outcomes (cognitive function) rather than clinical outcomes likely to be important to people with Alzheimer's disease and their carers.

OPTION GINKGO BILOBA

One systematic review of RCTs found good evidence that ginkgo biloba improves cognitive function and is well tolerated.

Benefits: One systematic review (search date 2000) identified nine double blind RCTs in people with Alzheimer's disease, vascular or mixed Alzheimer/vascular dementia.[20] Most of these trials were of short duration and used different entry criteria, outcomes, and dosage. Eight of these found that ginkgo biloba was superior to placebo for a variety of outcomes. The largest and longest trial (52 weeks; 309

people, of which 236 had Alzheimer's disease) found treatment in people with Alzheimer's disease to be significantly associated with improved ADAS-cog score (–1.7, 95% CI –3.2 to –0.2), GERRI (care giver assessed improvement, –0.19, 95% CI –0.28 to –0.08), but not in mean clinician's global impression of change (0, 95% CI –0.2 to +0.2).[20] The trial suffered from high withdrawal rate (137 withdrew); completer analysis for people with Alzheimer's disease or vascular dementia yielded the number needed to treat for a four point change in ADAS-cog at 8 (95% CI, 5 to 50).

Harms: The largest trial reported adverse events in 31% with ginkgo biloba versus 31% with placebo.[21] No specific pattern of adverse events was reported.

Comment: In the UK ginkgo biloba is currently classified as a foodstuff, and can be purchased freely. Manufacturers of ginkgo biloba sponsored all trials identified in the review. The high withdrawal rate of the longer RCT cited above weakens its conclusions, although the authors did conduct completer and intention-to-treat analysis.[21]

OPTION NON-STEROIDAL ANTI-INFLAMMATORY DRUGS

One small RCT found no benefit from diclofenac compared with placebo.

Benefits: We found no systematic review. We found one RCT comparing diclofenac plus misoprostol versus placebo for 25 weeks (41 people).[22] No significant differences were found between the groups, although for most outcome measures there was a trend to improvement in the NSAID arm, including ADAS-cog scores (mean difference 1.14, 95% CI –2.9 to +5.2) and clinician global impression of change (0.24, 95% CI–0.26 to 0.74).

Harms: Twelve (50%) participants in the treatment arm withdrew by week 25, compared with two in the placebo group. No serious drug related adverse events were reported.[22]

Comment: Inflammatory processes may play a part in the pathogenesis of Alzheimer's disease. However, despite the considerable interest in the putative role of NSAIDs, there is poor evidence at present to support the use of these drugs in Alzheimer's disease.

QUESTION What are the effects of non-drug treatments?

OPTION REMINISCENCE THERAPY

We found insufficient evidence on the effects of reminiscence therapy (see glossary, p 7) in people with dementia.

Benefits: We found one systematic review of reminiscence therapy (search date 1998), which identified two trials. Analysis of pooled data was compromised by poor trial methods and diverse outcomes.[23]

Harms: We found no evidence.

Comment: None.

OPTION REALITY ORIENTATION

One systematic review of small RCTs found that reality orientation (see glossary below) was associated with improved cognitive function and behaviour compared with no treatment. We found no data on adverse events.

Benefits: We found one systematic review (search date 1997, 6 RCTs, 125 people).[24] These compared reality orientation versus no treatment, using different measures of cognition. The review found that reality orientation improved cognitive function score (SMD –0.59, 95% CI –0.95 to –0.22) and behavioural symptom score (SMD –0.66, 95% CI –1.27 to –0.05).

Harms: The trials gave no information on adverse effects.[24]

Comment: The trials did not use standardised interventions or outcomes, and the review did not pool the data.[24]

GLOSSARY

Reality orientation Involves presenting information that is designed to reorient a person in time, place, or person. It may range in intensity from a board giving details of the day, date, and season, to staff reorienting a patient at each contact.
Reminiscence therapy Involves encouraging people to talk about the past in order to enable past experiences to be brought into consciousness. It relies on remote memory, which is relatively well preserved in mild to moderate dementia.

Substantive changes since last issue of Clinical Evidence

Cholinesterase inhibitors New systematic review found that rivastigmine improved cognitive function more than placebo in Alzheimer's disease.[13]

REFERENCES

1. Livingston G. The scale of the problem. In Burns A, Levy R, eds. *Dementia*. 1st ed. London: Chapman and Hall, 1994:21–35.
2. Panisset M, Stern Y, Gauthier S, eds. *Clinical diagnosis and management of Alzheimer's disease*, 1st ed. London: Dunitz, 1996:129–139.
3. McKeith I. The differential diagnosis of dementia. In: Burns A, Levy R, eds. *Dementia*, 1st ed. London: Chapman and Hall, 1994:39–57.
4. Hardy J. Molecular classification of Alzheimer's disease. *Lancet* 1991;i:1342–1343.
5. Eastwood R, Reisberg, B. Mood and behaviour. In: Panisset M, Stern Y, Gauthier S, eds. *Clinical diagnosis and management of Alzheimer's disease*, 1st ed. London: Dunitz, 1996:175–189.
6. Absher JR, Cummings JL. Cognitive and noncognitive aspects of dementia syndromes. In: Burns A, Levy R, eds. *Dementia*, 1st ed. London: Chapman and Hall, 1994:59–76.
7. Rosen WG, Mohs RC, Davis KL. A new rating scale for Alzheimer's disease. *Am J Psychiatry* 1984; 141:1356–1364.
8. Folstein MF, Folstein SE, McHugh PR. Mini Mental State: a practical method for grading the cognitive state of patients for the clinician. *J Psychiatr Res* 1975;12:189–198.
9. Birks JS, Melzer D. Donepezil for mild and moderate Alzheimer's disease. In: The Cochrane Library, Issue 2, 2000. Oxford: Update Software. Search date 1998; primary sources Cochrane Dementia and Cognitive Impairment Group Register of Clinical Trials, Medline, PsychLit, Embase and general contact with members of the Donepezil Study Group and Eisai Inc.
10. Rogers SL, Farlow MR, Doody RS, et al. A 24-week double blind placebo controlled trial of donepezil in patients with Alzheimer's disease. *Neurology* 1998;50:136–145.
11. Burns A, Rossor M, Gauthier S, et al. The effects of donezepil in Alzheimer's disease – results from a multinational trial. *Dementia Geriatr Disord* 1999;10:237–244.
12. Qizilbash N, Birks J, Lopez Arrieta J, et al. Tacrine in Alzheimer's disease. In: The Cochrane Library, Issue 2, 2000. Oxford: Update Software. Search date November 1998; primary sources the Cochrane Dementia Group Register of Clinical Trials.
13. Birks, J Iakovidou V, Tsolaki, M. Rivastigmine for Alzheimer's disease. In: The Cochrane Library, Issue 2, 2000. Oxford, Update Software. Search date 1999; primary sources Cochrane Controlled Trials Register, Cochrane Dementia Group Register of Clinical Trials, Medline, Embase, Psychlit, Cinahl, and hand searches of geriatric and dementia journals and conference abstracts.
14. Rosler M, Anand R, Cicin-Sain A. Efficacy and safety of rivastigmine in patients with Alzheimer's disease: international randomised controlled trial. *BMJ* 1999;318:633–640.
15. Knapp MJ, Knopman DS, Soloman PR, et al. A 30-week randomized controlled trial of high-dose tacrine in patients with Alzheimer's disease. *JAMA* 1994;271:985–991.
16. Kirchner V, Kelly C, Harvey R. Thioridazine for dementia. In: The Cochrane Library, Issue 2, 2000. Oxford: Update Software. Search date not given, amended August 1998; primary sources

Medline, Embase, Psychlit, Cinahl, Cochrane Group Register of Clinical Trials, and Novartis, the pharmaceutical company that develops and markets thioridazine was approached and asked to release any published or unpublished data they had on file.

17. Reilly JG, Ayis SA, Ferrier IN, et al. QT interval abnormalities and pychotropic drug therapy in psychiatric patients. Lancet 2000;355:1048–1052.
18. Birks J, Flicker L. Selegiline for Alzheimer's disease. In: The Cochrane Library, Issue 4, 1999. Oxford: Update Software. Search date not given, review amended August 1998; primary sources Cochrane Dementia and Cognitive Impairment Group Register of Clinical Trials.
19. Freedman M, Rewilak D, Xerri T, et al. L deprenyl in Alzheimer's disease. Cognitive and behavioural effects. *Neurology* 1998;50:660–668.
20. Ernst E, Pittler MH. Ginkgo biloba for dementia. *Clin Drug Invest* 1999;17:301–308. Search date 1998; primary sources Medline, Embase, Biosis, Cochrane Register of Controlled Clinical Trials, hand searches of bibliographies, and contact with manufacturers.
21. Le Bars P, Katz MM, Berman N, Itil T, Freedman A, Schatzberg. A placebo-controlled, double-blind, randomised trial of an extract of ginkgo biloba for dementia. *JAMA* 1997;278:1327–1332.
22. Scharf S, Mander A, Ugoni A, Vajda F, Christophidis N. A double-blind, placebo-controlled trial of diclofenac/misoprostol in Alzheimer's disease. *Neurology* 1999;53:197–201.
23. Spector A Orrell M. Reminiscence therapy for dementia. In: The Cochrane Library, Issue 4, 1999. Oxford: Update Software. Search date 1998; primary sources Cochrane Controlled Trials Register, Medline, Psychlit, Embase, Omni, Bids, Dissertation Abstracts International, Sigle, and reference lists of relevant articles, relevant internet sites, and hand searching of specialist journals.
24. Spector A, Orrell M, Davies S, et al. Reality orientation for dementia. In: The Cochrane Library, Issue 2, 2000. Oxford: Update Software. Search date 1997; primary sources Medline, Psychlit, Embase, Cochrane Database of Systematic Reviews, Omni, Bids, Dissertation Abstracts International, Sigle, plus Internet searching of HealthWeb, Mental Health Infosources, American Psychiatric Association, Internet Mental Health, Mental Health Net, NHS Confederation, and hand searching of specialist journals.

James Warner
Senior Lecturer/Consultant in Old Age Psychiatry
Imperial College School of Medicine
London
UK

Rob Butler
Lecturer in Old Age Psychiatry
Imperial College School of Medicine
London
UK

Competing interests: JW has been reimbursed by Novartis, the manufacturer of rivastigmine, for conference attendance. RB, none declared.

Anxiety disorder

Christopher Gale and Mark Oakley-Browne

QUESTIONS

INTERVENTIONS

Beneficial

Cognitive therapy 11

Likely to be beneficial

Buspirone. 14

Certain antidepressants (paroxetine, imipramine, trazodone, venlafaxine, mirtazepine) 15

Trade off between benefits and harms

Benzodiazepines 12

Unknown effectiveness

Applied relaxation 12

Antipsychotic drugs 16

β Blockers 16

To be covered in future issues of *Clinical Evidence*

Other antidepressants (amitriptyline, citalopram, monoamine oxidase inhibitors)

Barbiturates

Other non-drug treatments

Drug versus non-drug treatments

See glossary, p 17

Key Messages

Cognitive therapy

- Two systematic reviews of RCTs have found that cognitive therapy, with a combination of behavioural interventions such as exposure to anxiogenic circumstances, relaxation, and cognitive restructuring, is more effective than remaining on the waiting list, anxiety management training alone, or non-directive therapy. We found no evidence of adverse effects.

Applied relaxation

- One systematic review of RCTs comparing psychological treatments for generalised anxiety disorder has not established or excluded a clinically important difference in the effects of applied relaxation and cognitive therapy.

Benzodiazepines

- Two systematic reviews of RCTs have found that, compared with placebo, benzodiazepines are an effective and rapid treatment for generalised anxiety disorder (GAD). They increase the risk of dependence, sedation, industrial accidents and road traffic accidents. They have been associated with neonatal and infant morbidity when used late in pregnancy or while breast feeding. One RCT found no significant difference in the effects of slow release alprazolam and bromazepam.

Buspirone

- One systematic review has found that buspirone is effective in GAD. Limited evidence from RCTs found no significant difference in benefits between busipirone, benzodiazepines or antidepressants. Buspirone had slower onset than benzodiazepines but fewer adverse effects.

Antidepressants

- RCTs have found that imipramine, trazodone, venlafaxine, and paroxetine are effective treatments for GAD. One trial found that paroxetine was more effective than a benzodiazepine. Adverse effects of antidepressants include sedation, confusion, and falls.

Antipsychotic drugs

- One RCT in people with GAD found that trifluoperazine reduced anxiety more than placebo, but caused more adverse effects.

β Blockers

- We found that β blockers have not been adequately evaluated in GAD.

DEFINITION Generalised anxiety disorder (GAD) is defined as excessive worry and tension, on most days, for at least 6 months, together with the following symptoms and signs: increased motor tension (fatigability, trembling, restlessness, muscle tension); autonomic hyperactivity (shortness of breath, rapid heart rate, dry mouth, cold hands, and dizziness) but not panic attacks; and increased vigilance and scanning (feeling keyed up, increased startling, impaired concentration). One non-systematic review of epidemiological and clinical studies found marked reduction of quality of life and psychosocial functioning in people with anxiety disorder (including generalised anxiety disorder).[1] Significant impairment was also found in people with mild forms of anxiety disorders.[1]

INCIDENCE/ PREVALENCE Assessment of the incidence and prevalence of GAD is difficult. There is a high rate of comorbidity with other anxiety disorders and depressive disorders.[2] The reliability of the measures used in epidemiological studies is unsatisfactory.[3] One US study, which used the criteria of the Diagnostic and Statistical Manual of Mental Disorders, third edition, revised (DSM-III-R), has estimated that one in every 20 people will develop GAD at some time during their lives.[4] One recent non-systematic review found that the incidence of GAD in men is only half the incidence in women.[5] One non-systematic review of seven studies found reduced prevalence of anxiety disorders in older people.[6]

AETIOLOGY/ RISK FACTORS One small community study found that GAD was associated with an increase in the number of minor stressors, independent of demographic factors.[7] People with GAD complain of more somatic symptoms and respond in a rigid, stereotyped manner if placed under physiological stress. Autonomic function is similar to that of control populations, but muscle tension is increased.[8] One non-systematic review (five observational studies) of psychological sequelae to civilian trauma found rates of GAD reported in four of the five studies were increased significantly compared with a control population (rate ratio 3.3, 95% CI 2.0 to 5.5).[9]

PROGNOSIS GAD is a long term condition. It often begins before or during young adulthood and can be a lifelong problem. Spontaneous remission is rare.[4]

AIMS To reduce anxiety; to minimise disruption of day to day functioning; and to improve quality of life, with minimum adverse effects.

OUTCOMES Severity of symptoms and effects on quality of life, as measured by symptom scores, usually the Hamilton Anxiety Scale (HAM-A), State-Trait Anxiety Inventory (STAI), or clinical global impression symptom scores. Where NNTs are given, these represent the number of people requiring treatment within a given time period (usually 6–12 weeks) for one additional person to achieve a certain improvement in symptom score. The method for obtaining NNTs was not standardised across studies. Some used a reduction by, for example, 20 points in the HAM-A as a response, while others defined a response as a reduction, for example, by 50% of the premorbid score. We have not attempted to standardise methods but instead have used the response rates reported in each study to calculate NNTs. Similarly, we have calculated NNHs from original trial data.

METHODS *Clinical Evidence* update search and appraisal May 2000. Recent changes in diagnostic classification make it hard to compare older studies with more recent ones. In the earlier classification system, DSM-III-R, the diagnosis was made only in the absence of other psychiatric disorder. In current systems (DSM-IV and ICD-10 [International Classification of Diseases, 10th revision]), GAD can be diagnosed in the presence of any comorbid condition. All drug studies were short term, at most 12 weeks.

QUESTION What are the effects of cognitive therapy?

Two systematic reviews of RCTs have found that cognitive therapy, using a combination of behavioural interventions such as exposure, relaxation, and cognitive restructuring, is more effective than remaining on a waiting list (no treatment), anxiety management training alone, or non-directive therapy. We found no evidence of adverse effects.

Benefits: We found two systematic reviews. The first (search date 1996) included 35 RCTs (n = 4002 [60% women]) of medical treatment, cognitive therapy, or both.[10] Thirteen trials included 22 cognitive behavioural therapies, which involved (alone or in combination) cognitive restructuring, relaxation training, exposure, and systematic desensitisation. Combined results from these trials found significantly better results with active treatment compared with control treatments (effect size 0.70, 95% CI 0.57 to 0.83). Controls included remaining on a waiting list, anxiety management training, relaxation training, and non-directive psychotherapy. One year follow up of an RCT found cognitive therapy was associated with better outcomes than analytic psychotherapy and anxiety management training.[10,11] The second systematic review (search date 1998, 8 RCTs, n = 404) found that more participants given individual cognitive therapy maintained recovery after 6 months than those given other treatments (participants maintaining recovery at 6 months: individual cognitive therapy 41%, non-directive therapy 19%, group cognitive therapy 18%, group behaviour therapy 12%, individual behaviour therapy 18%, and analytical psychotherapy 0%; P values not reported).[12]

Harms: We found no evidence of adverse effects.

Comment: None.

QUESTION What are the effects of applied relaxation?

We found no study of applied relaxation (see glossary, p 17) versus placebo treatment. One systematic review of RCTs comparing applied relaxation with cognitive therapy found no significant difference in the proportion of people with clinically important improvement of their anxiety scores over 6 months. The available evidence does not establish or exclude the possibility of clinically important differences in the effects of applied relaxation and cognitive therapy.

Benefits: **Versus placebo:** We found no systematic review or RCT. **Versus other psychological treatments:** We found one systematic review (search date 1998, 6 RCTs, n = 404) of psychological therapy in GAD. The six RCTs all used the State-Trait Anxiety Inventory (STAI). There was significant variation in the type of cognitive therapy (group or individual) and in the comparison therapies (applied relaxation, analytical psychotherapy, behaviour therapy, and non-directive therapy). Only one of the six RCTs included a placebo group, and that RCT did not examine applied relaxation. Two RCTs included individual applied relaxation (n = 38) and four included individual cognitive behavioural therapy (n = 87). The systematic review analysed the raw data from individual studies to calculate the proportion of people who experienced a clinically significant change after treatment and maintained that improvement until 6 months after treatment. Applied relaxation was more likely than individual cognitive behavioural therapy to improve the anxiety inventory after 6 months (52% with applied relaxation *v* 41%).[12] No statistical tests of significance were performed by the systematic review, but even if the figures presented are taken at face value (see comment below) then the difference between the effects of individual applied relaxation and individual cognitive behavioural therapy may have arisen by chance (recovery maintained to 6 months: 20/38 = 52% with applied relaxation, 41/87 = 41% with cognitive therapy; RR 1.27, 95% CI 0.82 to 1.70).

Harms: No evidence of harms was noted.

Comment: The STAI covers only a restricted range of symptoms, and it may not satisfactorily reflect treatment outcomes in GAD. It is very difficult to interpret the results of the systematic review because the comparison involves arms from different RCTs. This could remove the benefits of randomisation because the groups being compared may have different characteristics. The figures presented in the systematic review produce estimates of relative effectiveness with wide confidence intervals: a clinically important difference has not been established or excluded.

QUESTION What are the effects of drug treatments?

OPTION BENZODIAZEPINES

One systematic review of RCTs has found that, compared with placebo, benzodiazepines are an effective and rapid treatment for GAD. They increase the risk of dependence, sedation, industrial accidents, and road traffic accidents. If used in late pregnancy or while breast feeding, they

can cause adverse effects in neonates. One RCT found no significant difference between sustained release alprazolam and bromazepam. One RCT found no evidence of a difference in effectiveness between benzodiazepines and buspirone. One systematic review of RCTs, which looked at long term treatment, found no good evidence that any short term benefit of benzodiazepines was sustained.

Benefits: **Versus placebo:** We found one systematic review (search date January 1996), which identified 24 placebo controlled trials of drug treatments, principally benzodiazepines (in 19 trials), buspirone (in nine trials), antidepressants (ritanserin and imipramine, in three trials), all in people with GAD.[10] Pooled analysis across all studies gave an effect size of 0.60 (95% CI 0.50 to 0.70), whereas for benzodiazepines the mean effect size was 0.70 (no 95% CIs given). The review found no significant differences in effect sizes between different benzodiazepines, although there was insufficient power to rule out a clinically important difference. One of the larger included trials (n = 230) found that the number of people reporting global improvement after 8 weeks (completer analysis, overall dropout rate 35%, no significant difference in withdrawal rates between groups) was greater with diazepam than with placebo (diazepam 67%, placebo 39%, $P < 0.026$). **Versus each other:** One subsequent RCT (n = 121) compared sustained release alprazolam with bromazepam and found no significant difference in effects (HAM-A scores).[13] **Versus buspirone:** See buspirone option, p 14. **Long term treatment:** We found one systematic review of eight RCTs (any benzodiazepine medication, greater than 2 months duration, people with GAD). The methods of these RCTs included limiting factors that prevent firm conclusions being made.[14]

Harms: **Sedation and dependence:** Benzodiazepines have been found to cause impairment in attention, concentration, and short term memory. One RCT found a high rate of drowsiness (71% with diazepam *v* 13% with placebo; $P = 0.001$) and dizziness (29% *v* 11%; $P = 0.001$).[10] Sedation can interfere with concomitant psychotherapy. Rebound anxiety on withdrawal has been reported in 15–30% of participants.[15] There is a high risk of substance abuse and dependence with benzodiazepines. **Memory:** Thirty one people with agoraphobia/panic disorder from a placebo controlled trial of 8 weeks' alprazolam were followed up at 3.5 years. Five were still taking benzodiazepines and had significant impairment in memory tasks.[16] There was no difference in memory performance between those who had been in the placebo group and those who had been given alprazolam but were no longer taking the drug. **Road traffic accidents:** We found one systematic review (search date 1997) examining the relation between benzodiazepines and road traffic accidents.[17] In the case control studies identified, the odds ratio for death or emergency medical treatment in those who had taken benzodiazepines compared with those who had not taken them ranged from 1.45 to 2.4. The odds ratio increased with higher doses and more recent intake. In the police and emergency ward studies, benzodiazepine use was a factor in 1–65% of accidents (usually 5–10%). In two studies in which participants had blood alcohol concentrations under the legal limit, benzodiazepines were found in 43% and 65%. For drivers over 65 years, the risk of being involved in reported road traffic accidents was higher if they had taken longer acting and larger quantities of benzodiazepines. These studies are retrospective case control studies and are therefore subject to confounding factors. **Pregnancy and breast feeding:** One systematic review (search date 1997) identified 23 studies looking at the link between cleft lip and palate and use of benzodiazepines in the first trimester of pregnancy.[18] The review found no association. However, use of benzodiazepines in late pregnancy has been found to be associated with neonatal hypotonia and withdrawal syndrome.[19] Benzodiazepines are secreted in breast milk, and there have been reports of sedation and hypothermia in infants.[19] **Other:** A reanalysis of eight RCTs of benzodiazepines compared with placebo or buspirone found a consistent improvement with benzodiazepines. However, recent use of benzodiazepines limited the effectiveness of buspirone.[20]

Comment: All the benzodiazepine studies were short term (at most 12 weeks). There was usually a significant improvement at 6 weeks, but response rates were given at the end of the trials.

OPTION BUSPIRONE

RCTs have found that, compared with placebo, buspirone increases the proportion of people with GAD who improve clinically in the short term. Limited evidence from RCTs found no significant differences in the benefits of buspirone, benzodiazepines or antidepressants. Buspirone had slower onset than benzodiazepines but had fewer adverse effects.

Benefits: **Versus placebo:** We found one systematic review (search date January 1996), which identified nine studies of buspirone but did not report on its effects as distinct from pharmacotherapy in general.[11] One of the included studies was itself a non-systematic meta-analysis of eight placebo controlled trials of buspirone in 520 people with GAD (see comment below). It found that, compared with placebo, buspirone was associated with a greater response rate, defined as the proportion of people much or very much improved as rated by their physician (54% *v* 28%, $P \leq 0.001$). A subsequent double blind placebo controlled trial in 162 people with GAD found similar results (buspirone 55% *v* placebo 35%, $P < 0.05$).[21] A reanalysis of pooled data from eight RCTs ($n = 735$) found a differential response to buspirone depending on whether the participant had been exposed to benzodiazepines (no previous exposure to benzodiazepine: response rate 62% [buspirone] *v* 31% [placebo]; recent benzodiazepine use: response rate 41% [buspirone] *v* 21% [placebo]). The latter result was not significant.[20] **Versus benzodiazepines:** The systematic review did not directly compare buspirone with benzodiazepines. One large RCT ($n = 230$) included in the review found no significant difference between buspirone and benzodiazepines.[10] A recent reanalysis of eight RCTs found no significant difference in the effects of buspirone compared with benzodiazepines.[20] **Versus antidepressants:** See antidepressants, p 15.

Harms: **Sedation and dependence:** The systematic review found that, compared with benzodiazepines, buspirone had a slower onset of action but fewer adverse effects.[10] The subsequent RCT found that, compared with placebo, buspirone caused significantly more nausea (34% v 13%), dizziness (64% v 12%), and somnolence (19% v 7%). We found no reports of dependency on buspirone. **Pregnancy and breast feeding:** We found no evidence.

Comment: All trials in the meta-analysis mentioned above were sponsored by pharmaceutical companies and had been included in new drug applications for buspirone as an antidepressant. Other search criteria were not given. Trial methods were similar.[10]

OPTION ANTIDEPRESSANTS

RCTs have found that imipramine, trazodone, venlafaxine, and paroxetine are effective treatments for GAD. Individual RCTs found that they were more effective than benzodiazepines, with no evidence of a difference in effectiveness compared with buspirone. There is a significant risk of sedation, confusion, and falls with these drugs.

Benefits: **Versus placebo:** We found one systematic review (search date January 1996, 3 placebo controlled RCTs) of antidepressants which found treatment to be significantly associated with a greater response than placebo (pooled effect size 0.57).[10] The review pooled results for trazodone, imipramine, and ritanserin, so limiting the conclusions that may be drawn for trazodone and imipramine alone.[10] In another placebo controlled RCT (n = 230) the NNT for moderate or pronounced improvement after 8 weeks of treatment with imipramine was 3 (completer analysis calculated from data by author) and with trazodone the NNT was 4 (95% CI 3 to 4, calculated from data by author).[22] **Versus benzodiazepines:** We found one RCT comparing paroxetine, imipramine, and 2'-chlordesmethyldiazepam for 8 weeks in 81 people with GAD.[23] Paroxetine and imipramine were significantly more effective than 2'-chlordesmethyldiazepam in improving anxiety scores (mean HAM-A after 8 weeks 11.1 for paroxetine, 10.8 for imipramine, 12.9 for 2'- chlordesmethyldiazepam; P = 0.05). **Versus buspirone:** We found no systematic review. We found one RCT (n = 365) comparing venlafaxine 75 mg and 150 mg/day with buspirone 30 mg/day over 8 weeks, with a small placebo arm. There was no significant difference between the two treatments (venlafaxine 75 mg, NNT 8, 95% CI 6 to 9; venlafaxine 150 mg, NNT 7, 95% CI 6 to 9; buspirone 30 mg, NNT 11, 95% CI 10 to 12).[24] **Sedating tricyclic antidepressants:** We found no systematic review or RCTs evaluating sedating tricyclics in people with GAD.

Harms: Sedation, confusion, dry mouth, and constipation have been reported with both imipramine and trazodone.[22] **Overdose:** In a series of 239 coroner directed necropsies from 1970 to 1989, tricyclic antidepressants were considered to be a causal factor in 12% of deaths and hypnosedatives (primarily benzodiazepines and excluding barbiturates) in 8%.[25] **Accidental poisoning:** From 1958 to 1977 a total of 598 deaths in British children under the age of 10 years were registered as accidental poisoning. After 1970, tricyclic antidepressants were the most common cause of accidental poisoning in this age group.[26] A study estimated that there was one death for every 44 children admitted to hospital after ingestion of tricyclic antidepressants.[27] **Hyponatraemia:** A case series reported 736 incidents of hyponatraemia in people taking selective serotonin reuptake inhibitors (SSRIs); 83% of episodes were in hospital inpatients aged over 65 years.[28] It is not possible to establish causation from this type of data. **Nausea:** Nausea has been reported in people taking paroxetine.[23] **Falls:** A retrospective cohort study of 2428 elderly residents of nursing homes found an increased risk of falls in new users of antidepressants (adjusted RR for tricyclic antidepressants: 2.0, 95 % CI 1.8 to 2.2, n = 665; for SSRIs: 1.8, 95% CI 1.6 to 2.0, n = 612; and for trazodone: 1.2, 95% CI 1.0 to 1.4, n = 304).[29] The increased rate of falls persisted through the first 180 days of treatment and beyond. A case control study of 8239 people aged 66 years or older treated in hospital for hip fracture found an increased risk of hip fracture in those taking antidepressants.[30] The adjusted odds ratio for hip fracture compared with those not taking antidepressants was 2.4 (95% CI 2.0 to 2.7) for SSRIs, 2.2 (95% CI 1.8 to 2.8) for secondary amine tricyclic antidepressants such as nortriptyline, and 1.5 (95% CI 1.3 to 1.7) for tertiary amine tricyclic antidepressants such as amitriptyline. This study could not control for confounding factors; people taking antidepressants may be at increased risk of hip fracture for other reasons. **In pregnancy:** We found no reports of harmful effects in pregnancy. One case controlled study found no evidence that imipramine or fluoxetine increased the rate of malformations in pregnancy.[31]

Comment: None.

OPTION ANTIPSYCHOTIC DRUGS

One RCT found that 4 weeks treatment with trifluoperazine lowered anxiety more than placebo but caused more adverse effects.

Benefits: We found no systematic review. We found one RCT (n = 415) comparing 4 weeks of treatment with trifluoperazine 2–6 mg/day with placebo in people with GAD.[32] The trial reported an average reduction of 14 points on the total anxiety rating scale (HAM-A), with no reduction on placebo ($P < 0.001$).

Harms: Short term treatment with antipsychotic drugs increased the risk of sedation, acute dystonias, akathisia, and parkinsonism. In the longer term, the rate of tardive dyskinesia may be increased, especially if treatment is interrupted.[33]

Comment: None.

OPTION β BLOCKERS

β Blockers have not been adequately evaluated in people with GAD.

Benefits: We found no systematic review or good RCTs of β blockers in people with GAD.

Harms: We found no good evidence in people with GAD.

Comment: None.

GLOSSARY

Applied relaxation A technique involving imagination of relaxing situations to induce muscular and mental relaxation.

Substantive changes since last issue of Clinical Evidence

Definition One non-systematic review has found that anxiety disorders compromise quality of life.[1]

Incidence and prevalence One non-systematic review found that men have half the incidence of GAD as women.[5] One non-systematic review found a decrease in the prevalence of anxiety disorders associated with increasing age.[6]

Aetiology/risk factors One non-systematic review of psychological sequelae to civilian trauma found rates of GAD were increased significantly.[9]

Cognitive behaviour One systematic review found that individual cognitive therapy was superior to other methods.[12]

Long term benzodiazepines One systematic review found no good evidence for an effective long term treatment.[15]

Harms from benzodiazepines A reanalysis of eight RCTs found recent benzodiazepine use was associated with an increase in nervousness and dizziness.[20]

Buspirone versus placebo A reanalysis of data from 8 RCTs found that previous exposure to benzodiazepines reduced the response to buspirone.[20]

Buspirone versus benzodiazepines A reanalysis of data from 8 RCTs found no difference in the effects of buspirone compared with benzodiazepine.[20]

REFERENCES

1. Mendlowicz MV, Stein MB. Quality of life in individuals with anxiety disorders. *Am J Psychiatry* 2000;157:669–682.
2. Judd LL, Kessler RC, Paulus MP, et al. Comorbidity as a fundamental feature of generalised anxiety disorders: results from the national comorbidity study (NCS). *Acta Psychiatr Scand* 1998;98(suppl 393):6–11.
3. Andrews G, Peters L, Guzman AM, Bird K. A comparison of two structured diagnostic interviews: CIDI and SCAN. *Aust N Z J Psychiatry* 1995;29:124–132.
4. Jessker RC, McGonagle KA, Zhao S, et al. Lifetime and 12-month prevalence of DSM-III-R psychiatric disorders in the United States: results from the national comorbidity survey. *Arch Gen Psychiatry* 1992;51:8–19.
5. Pigott T. Gendere differences in the epidemiology and treatment of anxiety disorders. *J Clin Psychiatry* 1999;60(suppl 18):15–18.
6. Jorm AF. Does old age reduce the risk of anxiety and depression? A review of epidemiological studies across the adult life span. *Psych Med* 2000;30:11–22.
7. Brantley PJ, Mehan DJ, Ames SC, Jones GN. Minor stressors and generalised anxiety disorders among low income patients attending primary care clinics. *J Nerv Ment Dis* 1999;187:435–440.
8. Hoehn-Saric R. Psychic and somatic anxiety: worries, somatic symptoms, and physiological changes. *Acta Psychiatr Scand* 1998;98(suppl 393):32–38.
9. Brown ES, Fulton MK, Wilkeson A, Petty F. The psychiatric sequelae of civilian trauma. *Comp Psychiatry* 2000;41:19–23.
10. Gould RA, Otto MW, Pollack MH, Yap L. Cognitive behavioural and pharmacological treatment of generalised anxiety disorder: a preliminary meta-analysis. *Behav Res Ther* 1997;28:285–305. Search date January 1996; primary sources Psyclit 1974 to 1996; Medline 1966 to January 1996; examination of reference lists; and unpublished articles presented at national conferences.
11. Durham RC, Fisher PL, Trevling LR, Hau CM, Richard K, Stewart JB. One year follow-up of cognitive therapy, analytic psychotherapy and anxiety management training for generalised anxiety disorder: symptom change, medication usage and attitudes to treatment. *Behav Cogn Psychother* 1999;27:19–35.
12. Fisher PL, Durham RC. Recovery rates in generalized anxiety disorder following psychological therapy: an analysis of clinically significant change in the STAI-T across outcome studies since 1990. *Psychol Med* 1999;29:1425–1434. Search date: December 1998; primary sources Medline 1987 to December 1998; Psychlit 1987 to December 1998; and Cochrane Controlled Trials Register 1987 to December 1998.
13. Figueira ML. Alprazolam SR in the treatment of generalised anxiety: a multicentre controlled study with bromazepam. *Hum Psychother* 1999;14: 171–177.
14. Mahe V, Balogh A. Long-term pharmacological treatment of generalized anxiety disorder. *Int Clin Psychopharmacol* 2000;15:99–105.
15. Tyrer P. Current problems with the benzodiazepines. In: Wheatly D, ed. *The anxiolytic jungle: where next?* Chichester: J Wiley and Sons, 1990;23–60.
16. Kilic C, Curran HV, Noshirvani H, Marks IM, Basoglu MB. Long-term effects of alprazolam on memory: a 3.5 year follow-up of agoraphobia/ panic patients. *Psychol Med* 1999;29:225–231.
17. Thomas RE. Benzodiazepine use and motor vehicle accidents. Systematic review of reported association. *Can Fam Physician* 1998;44:799–808. Search date 1997; primary sources Medline 1980 to 1997.
18. Dolovich LR, Addis A, Regis Vaillancourt JD, et al. Benzodiazepine use in pregnancy and major malformations of oral cleft: meta-analysis of cohort and case-control studies. *BMJ* 1998;317:

839–843. Search date December 1998; primary sources Medline 1966 to 1997; Embase 1980 to 1997; Reprotox, references of included studies and review articles.
19. Bernstein JG. *Handbook of drug therapy in psychiatry*, 3rd ed. St Louis, Missouri: Mosby Year Book, 1995:401.
20. DeMartinis N, Rynn M, Rickels K, Mandos L. Prior benzodiazepine use and buspirone response in the treatment of generalized anxiety disorder. *J Clin Psychiatry* 2000;61:91–94.
21. Sramek JJ, Transman M, Suri A, et al. Efficacy of buspirone in generalized anxiety disorder with coexisting mild depressive symptoms. *J Clin Psychiatry* 1996;57:287–291.
22. Rickels K, Downing R, Schweizer E, Hassman H. Antidepressants for the treatment of generalised anxiety disorder: a placebo-controlled comparison of imipramine, trazodone and diazepam. *Arch Gen Psychiatry* 1993;50:884–895.
23. Rocca P, Fonzo V, Scotta M, Zanalda E, Ravizza L. Paroxetine efficacy in the treatment of generalized anxiety disorder. *Acta Psychiatr Scand* 1997:95: 444–450.
24. Davidson JR, DuPont RL, Hedges D, Haskins JT. Efficacy, safety and tolerability of venlafaxine extended release and busperone in outpatients with generalised anxiety disorder. *J Clin Psychiatry* 1999;60:528–535.
25. Dukes PD, Robinson GM, Thomson KJ, Robinson BJ. Wellington coroner autopsy cases 1970–89: acute deaths due to drugs, alcohol and poisons. *N Z Med J* 1992;105:25–27. (Published erratum appears in *N A Med J* 1992;105:135.)
26. Fraser NC. Accidental poisoning deaths in British children 1958–77. *BMJ* 1980;280:1595–1598.
27. Pearn J, Nixon J, Ansford A, Corcoran A. Accidental poisoning in childhood: five year urban population study with 15 year analysis of fatality. *BMJ* 1984;288:44–46.
28. Lui BA, Mitmann N, Knowles SR, Shear NH. Hyponatremia and the syndrome of inappropriate secretion of antidiuretic hormone associated with the use of selective serotonin reuptake inhibitors: a review of spontaneous reports. *Can Med Assoc J* 1995;155:519–527.
29. Thapa PB, Gideon P, Cost TW, Milam AB, Ray WA. Antidepressants and the risk of falls among nursing home residents. *N Engl J Med* 1998;339: 875–882.
30. Liu B, Anderson G, Mittmann N, To T, Axcell T, Shear N. Use of selective serotonin-reuptake inhibitors of tricyclic antidepressants and risk of hip fractures in elderly people. *Lancet* 1998;351: 1303–1307.
31. Kulin NA, Pastuszak A, Koren G. Are the new SSRIs safe for pregnant women? *Can Fam Physician* 1998;44;2081–2083.
32. Mendels J, Krajewski TF, Huffer V, et al. Effective short-term treatment of generalized anxiety with trifluoroperazine. *J Clin Psychiatry* 1986;47:170–174.
33. Van Harten PN, Hoek HW, Matroos GE, Koeter M, Kahn RS. Intermittent neuroleptic treatment and risk of tardive dyskinesi: Curacao extrapyradimal syndromes study III. *Am J Psychiatry* 1998;155: 565–567.

Christopher Gale
Psychiatrist
Department of Psychiatry
University of Auckland
Auckland
New Zealand

Mark Oakley-Browne
Associate Professor
University of Auckland
Auckland
New Zealand

Competing interests: None declared.

Bulimia nervosa

Phillipa Hay and Josue Bacaltchuk

QUESTIONS

INTERVENTIONS

See glossary, p 25

Key Messages

Psychotherapy

- Two systematic reviews and a subsequent large RCT have found that cognitive behavioural therapy (CBT) reduces specific symptoms of bulimia nervosa and also improves non-specific symptoms, such as depression. One RCT found that the beneficial effects of CBT are maintained for at least 5 years.
- One systematic review of RCTs found that other psychotherapies improve the symptoms of bulimia nervosa.
- Two well designed RCTs found that the onset of the effects of interpersonal psychotherapy is slower than CBT.

Antidepressants

- Two systematic reviews of RCTs have found that antidepressants reduce bulimic symptoms in the short term, but we found insufficient evidence about their role in maintenance treatment.
- We found insufficient evidence about the effects of different classes of antidepressants.
- One systematic review of RCTs comparing antidepressants with psychotherapy found no significant difference in abstinence from binge eating.

Combinations of antidepressants and psychotherapy

- One systematic review of RCTs found that combinations of treatments are more effective than either individual psychotherapy or antidepressants alone. People taking antidepressants, either alone or in combination with psychotherapy, were more likely than people receiving psychotherapy alone to withdraw from treatment.

Bulimia nervosa

DEFINITION Bulimia nervosa is an intense preoccupation with body weight and shape, with regular episodes of uncontrolled overeating of large amounts of food (binge eating associated with use of extreme methods to counteract the feared effects of overeating). If a person also meets the diagnostic criteria for anorexia nervosa, then the diagnosis of anorexia nervosa takes precedence.[1] Bulimia nervosa can be difficult to identify because of extreme secrecy about binge eating and purgative behaviour. Weight may be normal but there is often a history of anorexia nervosa or restrictive dieting. Some people alternate between anorexia nervosa and bulimia nervosa.

INCIDENCE/ PREVALENCE In community based studies, the prevalence of bulimia nervosa is between 0.5% and 1.0%, with an even social class distribution.[2–4] About 90% of people diagnosed with bulimia nervosa are women. The numbers presenting with bulimia nervosa in industrialised countries increased during the decade that followed its recognition in the late 1970s and "a cohort effect" is reported in community surveys[2,5,6] implying an increase in incidence. The prevalence of eating disorders such as bulimia nervosa is lower in non-industrialised populations,[7] and varies across ethnic groups. African-American women have a lower risk of restrictive dieting than white American women, but have a similar risk of recurrent binge eating.[8]

AETIOLOGY/ RISK FACTORS Young women from the developed world who restrict their dietary intake are at highest risk of developing bulimia nervosa and other eating disorders. One community based case control study compared 102 people with bulimia nervosa with 204 healthy controls and found higher rates of the following in people with the eating disorder: obesity, mood disorder, sexual and physical abuse, parental obesity, substance misuse, low self esteem, perfectionism, disturbed family dynamics, parental weight/shape concern, and early menarche.[9] Compared to a control group of 102 women with other psychiatric disorders, women with bulimia nervosa had higher rates of parental problems and obesity.

PROGNOSIS A 10 year follow up study (50 people with bulimia nervosa from a former trial of mianserin treatment) found that 52% had fully recovered, and only 9% continued to experience symptoms of bulimia nervosa.[10] A larger study (222 people from a trial of antidepressants and structured intensive group psychotherapy) found that after a mean follow up of 11.5 years, 11% still met criteria for bulimia nervosa, while 70% were in full or partial remission.[11] Short term studies found similar results: about 50% of people made a full recovery, 30% made a partial recovery, and 20% continued to be symptomatic.[12] There are few consistent predictors of longer term outcome. Good prognosis has been associated with shorter illness duration, a younger age of onset, higher social class, and a family history of alcoholism.[10] Poor prognosis has been associated with a history of substance misuse,[11] premorbid and paternal obesity,[13] and, in some studies, personality disorder.[14–17]

AIMS To reduce symptoms of bulimia nervosa; to improve general psychiatric symptoms; to improve social functioning and quality of life.

OUTCOMES Frequency of binge eating, abstinence from binge eating, frequency of behaviours to reduce weight and counter the effects of binge eating, severity of extreme weight and shape preoccupation, severity of general psychiatric symptoms, severity of depression, improvement in social and adaptive functioning, remission rates, relapse rates, and withdrawal rates.

METHODS *Clinical Evidence* search and appraisal March 2000, and hand-search of reference lists of identified reviews. One RCT in press (since published) was identified through direct contact with an author.[18] One systematic review was not included as it included uncontrolled studies.[19]

QUESTION **What are the effects of treatments for bulimia nervosa in adults?**

OPTION **COGNITIVE BEHAVIOURAL THERAPY**

Two systematic reviews and one further large RCT have found that cognitive behavioural therapy (CBT) versus remaining on a waiting list reduces specific symptoms of bulimia nervosa, and improves non-specific symptoms, such as depression. Two RCTs found that CBT reduced binge eating in the short term more than interpersonal psychotherapy, but there was no significant difference in the long term.

Benefits: We found three systematic reviews of RCTs of psychotherapy[20–22] and two subsequent RCTs.[18,23] The third systematic review is in German and may be included in a future issue of *Clinical Evidence*.[22] The first systematic review (search date 1999, 20 RCTs) included RCTs of other binge eating disorders, although most studies were of people with bulimia nervosa (18 people with bulimia nervosa characterised by purging behaviour).[20] The second review (search date 1998, 26 RCTs) used a broad definition of CBT, including exposure and response prevention, and included non-randomised trials.[21] **Versus waiting list controls:** The first review (individual analyses included a maximum of 10 RCTs and 396 people) found that CBT compared to remaining on a waiting list increased the proportion of people abstaining from binge eating at the end of the trial (RR 0.64, 95% CI 0.53 to 0.78, 7 RCTs) (see table 1, p 27).[20] CBT compared with remaining on the waiting list was associated with lower depression scores (4 RCTs, 159 people). Weight at the end of treatment was similar with CBT and remaining on the waiting list (3 RCTs). There was insufficient evidence about other outcomes such as social functioning. The second systematic review (9 RCTs of specific CBT, 173 people) found that abstinence from binge eating at the end of treatment ranged from 33% to 92% (mean 55%).[21] Pooled effect sizes (weighted for sample size) ranged from 1.22 to 1.35 for reduction in binge eating frequency, purging frequency, depression, and disturbed eating attitudes. Tests for heterogeneity were not significant. In one study the benefits of CBT were maintained for up to 5 years.[13] **Versus other psychotherapies:** The first review found that more people abstained from binge eating after CBT than after other psychotherapies, but the difference was not significant (6 RCTs; RR 0.79, 95% CI 0.54 to 1.17).[20] CBT in a full or less intensive form was not significantly superior to CBT in a pure self help form (RR 0.94, 95% CI 0.76 to

1.17, 3 trials). CBT was associated with significantly lower depression scores at end of treatment compared with other psychotherapies (SMD –0.52, 95% CI –0.76 to –0.27, 8 RCTs, 273 people). CBT plus exposure therapy was not more effective than CBT alone (RR abstinence from binge eating 0.87, 95% CI 0.65 to 1.16, 4 RCTs). Depression scores were lower at the end of treatment in groups treated with CBT plus exposure therapy than in groups treated with CBT alone (SMD 0.54, 95% CI 0.17 to 0.91, 3 RCTs, 122 people). The first subsequent RCT compared classic CBT for bulimia nervosa with interpersonal psychotherapy in 220 people with bulimia nervosa that involved purging.[18] The trial found that CBT improved abstinence from binge eating at the end of treatment (intention to treat analysis: 29% with CBT *v* 6% with interpersonal psychotherapy). The differences were not significant at 4, 8, and 12 months' follow up. The benefit of CBT was established fully at the end of treatment and was maintained for up to 1 year. The benefits of interpersonal psychotherapy continued to improve in the year after treatment. The second subsequent RCT compared four sessions of motivational enhancement therapy versus CBT in 125 people with bulimia nervosa. The trial found no significant differences between the treatments.[23] **Versus antidepressants:** See antidepressants option, p 23.

Harms: The RCTs did not report details of the adverse effects.[18,20,21,23] One systematic review found no significant difference in completion rates between interventions,[20] suggesting no major difference in acceptability. However, neither review could exclude infrequent serious adverse effects. An observational study found that group psychotherapy offered very soon after presentation was sometimes perceived as threatening.[10]

Comment: The first review defined CBT as psychotherapy that uses specified techniques and models,[20] but it did not define the number of sessions or specialist expertise.[24] Effect sizes for CBT were large, but over 50% of people were still binge eating at the end of treatment.[20,21] Research is needed to evaluate the specific as well as non-specific effects of CBT and other psychotherapies, to identify individual characteristics that may predict response, and to explore the long term effects of treatment. Rates of abstinence from binge eating were higher in all experimental groups, but the differences reached significance only when compared with those remaining on a waiting list. It is difficult to interpret the clinical importance of the statistically significant changes in depression scores. It is also difficult to interpret directly the clinical importance of the benefits reported as effect sizes, where the individual RCTs used different outcomes. Further limitations are that the quality of trials was variable (e.g. 57% were not blinded and only one was truly double blinded).[20] Sample sizes were often small. None of the studies measured harms rigorously.

OPTION OTHER PSYCHOTHERAPIES

Two systematic reviews and one additional RCT have found that non-CBT psychotherapy increases abstinence from binge eating compared with waiting list controls.

Benefits: **Versus waiting list controls:** We found two systematic reviews of psychotherapy,[20,21] and one additional RCT.[25] The first review also included data from studies of other binge eating syndromes, and found that non-CBT psychotherapies (e.g. hypnobehavioural therapy and interpersonal psychotherapy) were associated with significantly greater abstinence rates compared with waiting list controls (RR 0.67, 95% CI 0.56 to 0.81, 3 RCTs, 131 people) and a greater reduction in bulimia nervosa symptom severity measures (SMD –1.2, 95% CI –1.52 to –0.87, 4 RCTs, 177 people). The additional small RCT (17 people with bulimia nervosa) compared structured, behaviour orientated group treatment with a waiting list. The trial found psychotherapy reduced binge eating frequency, depression, and other indices of eating disorder symptom severity.[25]

Harms: The RCTs did not report details of individual adverse events (see harms of cognitive behavioural therapy, p 22). Non-CBT psychotherapies include a large number of options, and it remains to be elucidated which therapies are most effective.

Comment: The quality of trials was variable, few were blinded, sample sizes were small, and none of the studies measured harms rigorously (see comment under cognitive behavioural therapy, p 22).

OPTION ANTIDEPRESSANTS

Two systematic reviews of RCTs have found short term reduction of bulimic symptoms and a small reduction of depressive symptoms. We found insufficient evidence about the persistence of these effects or about the effects of different classes of antidepressants. One systematic review of RCTs comparing antidepressants versus psychotherapy found no significant difference in abstinence from binge eating.

Benefits: We found two systematic reviews,[21,26] two additional RCTs,[27,28] and one subsequent RCT.[29] **Versus placebo:** Both reviews found that antidepressants reduced bulimic symptoms. The first review (search date 1998, 9 RCTs) found that antidepressants versus placebo significantly reduced binge eating (5 RCTs, 163 people; at the end of the trials 16% not binge eating with antidepressants; effect size weighted for sample size 0.66, 95% CI 0.52 to 0.81).[21] Antidepressants versus placebo improved purging (6 RCTs; effect size 0.39, 95% CI 0.24 to 0.54), depression (effect size 0.73, 95% CI 0.58 to 0.88), and improved scales of eating attitudes. The second review (search date 1997, 8 placebo controlled RCTs) found more frequent remission of bulimic episodes with antidepressants (19% *v* 8% with placebo; pooled RR 0.88, 95% CI 0.83 to 0.94; NNT 9, 95% CI 6 to 16). The review found no significant difference in effect between different classes of antidepressants, but there were too few trials to exclude a clinically important difference (see table 2, p 27). Fluoxetine was the only selective serotonin reuptake inhibitor (SSRI) included in the review, and only one trial reported remission rates.[26] Two additional RCTs (not in either of the above reviews) found a high relapse rate (30–45%) over 4–6 months.[27,28] Improvement was maintained after withdrawal of treatment that had been continued for 6 months.[30] The subsequent double blind RCT compared fluvoxamine versus placebo.[29] Relapse rates during a 15 week maintenance period after successful psychotherapy treatment were significantly higher applying an intention to treat analysis for placebo, but withdrawal rates were very high (19/33 people randomised to fluvoxamine). Fluvoxamine was associated with fewer relapses of general psychiatric symptoms and depression, but differences were not significant ($P < 0.1$).[31] **Versus CBT:** See benefits of cognitive behavioural therapy, p 21. **Versus psychotherapy:** We found one systematic review (5 RCTs) of antidepressants versus psychotherapy (all CBT trials) that found no significant difference in remission rates (39% with psychotherapies, 20% with antidepressants; effect size 1.28; $P = 0.07$), bulimic symptom severity (3 RCTs), or depression symptom severity at the end of the trial (3 RCTs).[25,32] **Antidepressants plus psychotherapy:** See benefits of combination treatment, p 25.

Harms: One systematic review found higher withdrawal rates with antidepressants than with psychotherapy (40% *v* 18%, 4 trials, 189 people, RR = 2.18, 95% CI 1.09 to 4.35).[33] The second systematic review found significantly higher withdrawal rates in people with bulimia taking antidepressants than with placebo (12 RCTs, 10.5% *v* 5.1%).[26] The review found no significant difference in withdrawal rates due to adverse effects among and within classes of antidepressants. In pooled analysis, withdrawal due to any cause was more likely with tricyclic antidepressants than with placebo (6 RCTs, 29% *v* 14.4%, $P = 0.01$), but more likely with placebo than SSRIs (3 RCTs, 37% *v* 40%, $P = 0.04$). We found two RCTs that examined specific adverse effects. One found significant increases in reclining and standing blood pulse rate, lying systolic and diastolic blood pressure, and greater orthostatic effects on blood pressure with desipramine than with placebo.[33] The cardiovascular changes were well tolerated, and few people withdrew because of these effects. Meta-analysis of two double blind RCTs of fluoxetine versus placebo found no significant difference in the incidence of suicidal acts or ideation in people treated with fluoxetine versus placebo.[34] However, the overall incidence of events was low (suicide attempts: 1.2%, none fatal; emergent suicidal ideation: 3.1%).

Comment: We found no consistent predictors of response to treatment. Antidepressants included in the trials were imipramine, amitriptyline, desipramine, phenylzine, isocaboxazid, brofaramine, fluoxetine, mianserin, and buproprion. We found no good evidence on the effects of newer antidepressants, such as venlafaxine and moclobemide. Both reviews commented on the lack of follow up.[21,26]

OPTION COMBINATION TREATMENT

One systematic review of RCTs has found that combination treatment (antidepressants plus psychotherapy) reduces binge frequency and increases rates of remission from binge eating more than either

intervention alone. Reporting of other outcome measures was poor. Antidepressants alone or in combination with psychotherapy were associated with higher withdrawal rates.

Benefits: We found one systematic review (search date 1997) comparing combination treatment (antidepressants plus psychotherapy) versus either treatment alone.[35] One meta-analysis compared antidepressants versus a combination of psychotherapy plus antidepressants.[35] Combined treatment was associated with significantly greater improvement in binge frequency and depressive symptoms (3 trials, effect size 0.47, P = 0.04), but there was no significant difference in rates of short term remission compared with antidepressants alone (4 RCTs, 141 people, 42% *v* 23%, RR 1.38, P = 0.06). A second meta-analysis compared psychotherapy alone versus a combination of psychotherapy plus antidepressants.[35] Combination treatment was associated with significantly higher rates of short term remission (6 RCTs, 257 people, 49% *v* 36%, RR 1.21, P = 0.03) and greater improvement in depressive symptoms, but no significant difference in frequency of binge eating compared with psychotherapy alone.

Harms: Withdrawal rates were lower after psychotherapy plus antidepressants than with antidepressants alone (4 trials, 196 people, 34% *v* 41%, RR 1.19, 95% CI 0.69 to 2.05).[35] Withdrawal rates were significantly higher with psychotherapy plus antidepressants than with psychotherapy alone (6 trials, 295 people, 30% *v* 16%, RR 0.57, P = 0.01).[35]

Comment: None.

GLOSSARY

Bulimia nervosa The American Psychiatric Association DSM-IV[1] criteria include recurrent episodes of binge eating; recurrent inappropriate compensatory behaviour to prevent weight gain; frequency of binge eating and inappropriate compensatory behaviour both, on average, at least twice a week for 3 months; self evaluation unduly influenced by body shape and weight; and disturbance occurring not exclusively during episodes of anorexia nervosa.

Types of bulimia nervosa, modified from DSM-IV[1]: purging: using self induced vomiting, laxatives, diuretics, or enemas. Non-purging: fasting, exercise, but not vomiting or other abuse as purging type.

Binge eating Modified from DSM-IV.[1] Eating, in a discrete period (e.g. hours), a large amount of food, and a sense of lack of control during the episode.

REFERENCES

1. American Psychiatric Association. *Diagnostic and statistical manual of mental disorders* 4th ed. Washington DC: American Psychiatric Press, 1994.
2. Bushnell JA, Wells JE, Hornblow AR, Oakley-Brown MA, Joyce P. Prevalence of three bulimic syndromes in the general population. *Psychol Med* 1990;20:671–680.
3. Garfinkel PE, Lin B, Goering P, et al. Bulimia nervosa in a Canadian community sample: Prevalence, co-morbidity, early experiences and psychosocial functioning. *Am J Psychiatry* 1995; 152:1052–1058.
4. Gard MCE, Freeman CP. The dismantling of a myth: A review of eating disorders and socioeconomic status. *Int J Eat Disord* 1996;20: 1–12.
5. Hall A, Hay PJ. Eating disorder patient referrals from a population region 1977–1986. *Psychol Med* 1991;21:697–701.
6. Kendler KS, Maclean C, Neale M, et al. The genetic epidemiology of bulimia nervosa *Am J Psychiatry* 1991;148:1627–1637.
7. Choudry IY, Mumford DB. A pilot study of eating disorders in Mirpur (Pakistan) using an Urdu version of the Eating Attitude Test. *Int J Eat Disord* 1992;11:243–251.
8. Striegel-Moore RH, Wifley DE, Caldwell MB, Needham ML, Brownell KD. Weight-related attitudes and behaviors of women who diet to lose weight: A comparison for black dieters and white dieters. *Obes Res* 1996;4:109–116.
9. Fairburn CG, Welch SL, Doll HA, Davies BA, O'Connor ME. Risk factors for bulimia nervosa: A community-based case-control study. *Arch Gen Psychiatry* 1997;54:509–517.

10. Collings S, King M. Ten year follow-up of 50 patients with bulimia nervosa. *Br J Psychiatry* 1994;164:80–87.
11. Keel PK, Mitchell JE, Miller KB, Davis TL, Crow SJ. Long-term outcome of bulimia nervosa. *Arch Gen Psychiatry* 1999;56:63–69.
12. Keel PK, Mitchell JE. Outcome in bulimia nervosa. *Am J Psychiatry* 1997;154:313–321.
13. Fairburn CG, Norman PA, Welch SL, et al. A prospective study of outcome in bulimia nervosa and the long-term effects of three psychological treatments. *Arch Gen Psychiatry* 1995;52:304–312.
14. Coker S, Vize C, Wade T, Cooper PJ. Patients with bulimia nervosa who fail to engage in cognitive behaviour therapy. *Int J Eat Disord* 1993;13:35–40.
15. Fahy TA, Russell GFM. Outcome and prognostic variables in bulimia. *Int J Eat Disord* 1993;14:135–146.
16. Rossiter EM, Agras WS, Telch CF, Schneider JA. Cluster B personality disorder characteristics predict outcome in the treatment of bulimia nervosa. *Int J Eat Disord* 1993;13:349–358.
17. Johnson C, Tobin DL, Dennis A. Differences in treatment outcome between borderline and nonborderline bulimics at 1-year follow-up. *Int J Eat Disord* 1990;9:617–627.
18. Agras WS, Walsh BT, Fairburn CG, Wilson GT, Kraemer HC. A multicenter comparison of cognitive-behavioral therapy and interpersonal psychotherapy. *Arch Gen Psychiatry* 2000;54:459–465.
19. Lewandowski LM, Gebing TA, Anthony JL, O'Brien WH. Meta-analysis of cognitive behavioural treatment studies for bulimia. *Clin Psychol Rev* 1997;17:703–718. Search date 1995; primary sources Psyinfo and hand searches of references lists.
20. Hay, PJ, Bacaltchuk J. Psychotherapy for bulimia nervosa and binging. In: The Cochrane Library, Issue 4, 1999. Oxford: Update software. Search dates 1999. Handsearch of *Int J Eat Disord* since its first issue; Medline 1966 to 1998; an Extramed, Embase, Psychlit, Current Contents, Lilacs, Scisearch up to 1998; the Cochrane Collaboration Controlled Trials Register 1997 Internet version; and the Cochrane Collaboration Depression and Anxiety Trials Register up to February 1999; handsearch of all citation lists in identified studies and reviews and personal contact.
21. Whittal ML, Agras WS, Gould RA. Bulimia nervosa: A meta-analysis of psychosocial and pharmacological treatments. *Behavr Ther* 1999; 30:117–135. Search dates "to present": presumed 1998 (date of submission); Psyclit 1974–1998; Medline 1966–1998; handsearch of *Int J Eat Disord* 1990–1998; handsearch other relevant (not specified) journals and identified studies. This was reviewed in Waller G. *Evidenced Based Medicine* (September/October 1999).
22. Jacobi C, Dahme B, Rustenbach S. Vergleich kontrollierter Psycho- und Pharmakaotherapiestudien bei Bulimia und Anorexia nervosa. *Psychother Psychosom Med Psychol* 1997;47:346–364. Search dates from 1994; Psych Abstracts, Medline, Psychindex, Psychinfo.
23. Treasure JL, Katzman M, Schmidt U, et al. Engagement and outcome in the treatment of bulimia nervosa: first phase of a sequential design comparing motivation enhancement therapy and cognitive behavioural therapy. *Behav Res Ther* 1999;37:405–418.
24. Wilson GT, Fairburn CG. Treatments for eating disorders. In Nathan PE, Gorman JM, eds. *A Guide to Treatments that Work*. New York: Oxford University Press, 1998:501–530.
25. Laessle RG, Waadt S, Pirke KM. A structured behaviourally orientated group treatment for bulimia nervosa. *Psychother Psychosom* 1987;48:141–145.
26. Bacaltchuk J, Hay P, Mari JJ. Antidepressants versus placebo for the treatment of bulimia nervosa: A systematic review. *Aust N Z J Psychiatry* 2000;34:310–317. Search dates 1997; handsearch of *Int J Eat Disord* since its first issue; Medline 1966–1998; an Extramed, Embase, Psychlit, Current Contents, Lilacs, Scisearch up to 1997; the Cochrane Collaboration Controlled Trials Register 1997 Internet version; and the Cochrane Collaboration Depression and Anxiety Trials Register; handsearch of all citation lists in identified studies and reviews and personal contact.
27. Walsh BT, Hadigan CM, Devlin MJ, Gladis M, Roose SP. Long-term outcome of antidepressant treatment for bulimia nervosa. *Am J Psychiatry* 1991;148:1206–1212.
28. Pyle RL, Mitchell JE, Eckert ED, et al. Maintenance treatment and 6-month outcome for bulimic patients who respond to initial treatment. *Am J Psychiatry* 1990;147:871–875.
29. Fichter MM, Kr ger R, Rief W, Holland R, Döhne J. Fluvoxamine in prevention of relapse in bulimia nervosa: effects on eating specific psychopathology. *J Clin Psychopharmacol* 1996; 16:9–18.
30. Agras WS, Rossiter EM, Arnow B, et al. One-year follow-up of psychosocial and pharmacologic treatments for bulimia nervosa *J Clin Psychiatry* 1994;55:179–183.
31. Fichter MM, Leibl C, Kr ger R, Rief W. Effects of fluvoxamine on depression, anxiety, and other areas of general psychopathology in bulimia nervosa. *Pharmacopsychiatry* 1997;30:85–92.
32. Bacaltchuk J, Trefiglio RP, de Oliveira IR, Lima MS, Mari JJ. Antidepressants versus psychotherapy for bulimia nervosa: a systematic review. *J Clin Pharm Ther* 1999;24:23–31. Search dates 1997; handsearch of *Int J Eat Disord* since its first issue; Medline 1966–1998; an Extramed, Embase, Psychlit, Current Contents, Lilacs, Scisearch up to 1997; Cochrane Collaboration Controlled Trials Register 1997 Internet version; Cochrane Collaboration Depression and Anxiety Trials Register; handsearch of all citation lists in identified studies and reviews and personal contact.
33. Agras WS, Rossiter EM, Arnow B, et al. Pharmacologic and cognitive-behavioral treatment for bulimia nervosa: A controlled comparison. *Am J Psychiatry* 1992;149:82–87. Cited in reference 28.
34. Wheadon DE, Rampey AH, Thompson VL, et al. Lack of association between fluoxetine and suicidality in bulimia nervosa. *J Clin Psychiatry* 1992;53:235–241.
35. Bacaltchuk J, Trefiglio RP, Oliveira IR, et al. Combination of antidepressants and psychotherapy for bulimia nervosa: a systematic review. *Acta Psychiatr Scand* 2000;101:256–264. Search dates 1997; handsearch of *Int J Eat Disord* since its first issue; Medline 1966–1998; an Extramed, Embase, Psychlit, Current Contents, Lilacs, Scisearch up to 1997; Cochrane Collaboration Controlled Trials Register 1997 Internet version; Cochrane Collaboration Depression and Anxiety Trials Register; handsearch of all citation lists in identified studies and reviews and personal contact.

Bulimia nervosa

Phillipa Hay
Psychiatrist
University of Adelaide
Adelaide
Australia

Josue Bacaltchuk
Psychiatrist
Federal University of Sao Paulo
Sao Paulo
Brazil

Competing interests: PH has received support to attend conferences and meetings from Pfizer PTY LTD, Solvay Pharmaceuticals, and Bristol-Myers Squibb Pharmaceuticals. JB has received fees from Janssen-Cilag Farmaceutica, Brazil.

TABLE 1 Comparison of remission rates between cognitive behaviour therapy (CBT) or other active psychotherapy and comparison group (see text, p 21).[20]

Comparison	Number of RCTs	N	Absolute remission rates	RR (95% CI)
CBT *v* waiting list	7	300	42% *v* 6%	0.64 (0.53 to 0.78)
CBT *v* other psychotherapy	7	474*	40% *v* 21%	0.80 (0.61 to 1.04)
CBT *v* pure self help CBT	3	183	45% *v* 37%	0.92 (0.48 to 1.77)
Other psychotherapy *v* waiting list	3	131	36% *v* 3%	0.67 (0.56 to 0.81)

*Updated to include new trial;[18] CBT, cognitive behavioural therapy.
N, number of participants.

TABLE 2 Comparison of remission rates between active drug and placebo by class of antidepressant (see text, p 23).[26]

Class: Drug(s)	Number of RCTs	N	RR	95% CI
TCA: desipramine, imipramine	3	132	0.86	0.7 to 1.07
SSRI: fluoxetine	1	398	0.92	0.84 to 1.01
	2	98	0.81	0.68 to 0.96
Other: bupropion, trazodone	2	87	0.86	0.76 to 0.97

MAOI, monoamine oxidase inhibitor; N, number of participants; SSRI, selective serotonin reuptake inhibitor; TCA, tricyclic antidepressant.

Depressive disorders

John Geddes, Rob Butler and James Warner

QUESTIONS

INTERVENTIONS

To be covered in future issues of *Clinical Evidence*
Behaviour therapy
Treatment for bipolar affective disorder

See glossary, p 39

Key Messages

- Systematic reviews of RCTs have found that antidepressant drugs are effective in acute treatment of all grades of depressive disorders in all common treatment settings and in people with or without coexistent physical illness. We found no evidence of a clinically significant difference in the benefits of different antidepressant drugs, although drugs vary in adverse effects.
- One systematic review of RCTs has found that cognitive therapy is effective and may be more effective than drug treatment for mild to moderate depression.
- One systematic review of mixed quality RCTs has found that St John's Wort is an effective treatment for mild to moderate depression.
- One large RCT has found that interpersonal therapy is effective treatment for mild to moderate depression. Less robust RCTs have found that problem solving therapy is also effective. Specific psychological treatments, such as cognitive and interpersonal therapy have been shown to be as effective as drugs.

- We found limited evidence suggesting that other treatments, including exercise, bibliotherapy, befriending, and non-directive counselling, may be effective.
- We found no reliable evidence to suggest that one type of treatment (drug or non-drug) is superior to another. Limited evidence suggests that combining drug and psychological treatments may be effective in severe but not mild to moderate depression.
- Of the interventions examined in this issue, prescription antidepressant drugs are the only treatment for which there is good evidence of effectiveness in severe and psychotic depressive disorders. We found no RCTs comparing drug and non-drug treatments in severe depressive disorder.
- RCTs have found that continuing antidepressant drug treatment for 4–6 months after recovery reduces risk of relapse.
- We found no evidence of a difference between treatments in terms of long term benefits.

DEFINITION Depressive disorders are characterised by persistent low mood, loss of interest and enjoyment, and reduced energy. They often impair function. **Older adults:** Older adults are generally defined as people aged 65 years or more. The presentation of depression in older adults may be atypical; low mood may be masked and anxiety or memory impairment may be the principal presenting symptoms. Dementia should be considered in the differential diagnosis of depression in older adults.[1]

INCIDENCE/ PREVALENCE **Younger adults:** Depressive disorders are common, with a prevalence of major depression between 5–10% of people seen in primary care settings.[2] Two to three times as many people may have depressive symptoms but do not meet criteria for major depression. Women are affected twice as often as men. Depressive disorders are the fourth most important cause of disability worldwide and are expected to become the second most important cause by 2020.[3,4] **Older adults:** 10–15% of older people have significant depressive symptomatology, although major depression is relatively rare in older adults.[5]

AETIOLOGY/ RISK FACTORS The causes are uncertain but include both childhood events and current psychosocial adversity.

PROGNOSIS About half of people suffering a first episode of major depressive disorder experience further symptoms in the next 10 years.[6] Different levels of severity[7,8] indicate different prognosis and treatment. **Mild to moderate depression** is characterised by depressive symptoms and some functional impairment. Many people recover in the short term but about half experience recurrent symptoms. **Severe depression** is characterised by additional agitation or psychomotor retardation with marked somatic symptoms. In this review, treatments are considered to have been evaluated in severe depression if the RCTs included inpatients. **Psychotic depression** is characterised by additional hallucinations, delusions, or both. **Older adults:** The prognosis may be especially poor in elderly people with a chronic or relapsing course.[9]

AIMS To improve mood, social and occupational functioning, and quality of life; to reduce morbidity and mortality; to prevent recurrence of depressive disorder; and to minimise adverse effects of treatment. Depression should not be regarded as a natural concomitant of older age.

OUTCOMES Depressive symptoms rated by the depressed person and clinician, social functioning, occupational functioning, quality of life, admission to hospital, rates of self harm, relapse of depressive symptoms, rates of adverse events. Trials often use continuous scales to measure depressive symptoms (such as the Hamilton Depression Rating Scale and the Beck Depression Inventory). Clinician reports and self reported global outcome measures are also used. Changes in continuous measures can be dealt with in two ways. They can be dichotomised in an arbitrary but clinically helpful manner (e.g. taking a reduction in depressive symptoms of more than 50% as an end point), which allows results to be expressed as relative risks and numbers needed to treat. Alternatively, they can be treated as continuous variables, as is done for systematic analysis. In this case, the pooled estimate of effect (the effect size) expresses the degree of overlap between the range of scores in the control and experimental groups. The effect size can be used to estimate the proportion of people in the control group who had a poorer outcome than the average person in the experimental group. **Older adults:** The Hamilton Depression Rating Scale is not ideal for older people because it includes a number of somatic items that may be positive in older people who are not depressed. It has been the most widely used scale, although specific scales for elderly people (such as the Geriatric Depression Scale) avoid somatic items.

METHODS A validated search for systematic reviews and RCTs was conducted between May and September 1998 from the Cochrane Database of Systematic Reviews and the Database of Abstract of Reviews of Effectiveness, *Best Evidence* and *Evidence-Based Mental Health*, Medline, PsychLit, and Embase. Studies were included by using epidemiological criteria and relevance to the clinical question. A *Clinical Evidence* update search and appraisal was conducted in May 2000 including a search for data on depression in older adults. To date, few studies have concentrated on older adults as a separate subgroup. Most published evidence for the efficacy of antidepressants includes all ages over 16 or is limited to people aged under 65.

QUESTION What are the effects of treatments?

OPTION PRESCRIPTION ANTIDEPRESSANT DRUGS

Younger adults: Systematic reviews of RCTs have found that antidepressant drugs are effective in acute treatment of all grades of depressive disorders. They have also found no clinically significant difference in effectiveness between different kinds of antidepressant drug. However, the drugs differ in their adverse event profiles. On average, people seem to tolerate selective serotonin reuptake inhibitors

(SSRIs) a little more than older drugs, but this difference is too small to be grounds for a policy of always choosing an SSRI as first line treatment. We found no strong evidence that fluoxetine is associated with increased risk of suicide. Abrupt withdrawal of SSRIs is associated with symptoms, including dizziness and rhinitis in some patients, and this is more likely and probably more severe with drugs with a short half life, such as paroxetine. Older adults: One systematic review has found that heterocyclic antidepressants and SSRIs are effective in older people with mild to moderate depression. However, overall treatment effects were modest. Limitations of this review include the variety of populations studied and the short duration of many studies. Future, high quality RCTs are unlikely for ethical reasons.

Benefits: **In younger adults: Versus placebo:** We found two systematic reviews.[10,11] The first review (published in 1996, search date not given, 49 RCTs in people with depressive disorder) included five trials of people admitted to hospital (probably more severely ill); 40 RCTs in a setting outside hospital; one in both settings; and three trials that did not specify the setting. Each RCT compared two antidepressant drugs and included a placebo control group. The review found a mean effect size of 0.50 for antidepressant drugs versus placebo, which means that 69% of those taking placebo did worse than the average person taking antidepressants. Drugs were more effective in those with depressive disorders diagnosed according to standard criteria (mainly *Diagnostic and Statistical Manual of Mental Disorders*, 3rd edition, revised [DSM-III-R]). The second systematic review (updated in 1998, 15 RCTs, 1871 people) compared antidepressant versus placebo in people with dysthymia (chronic mild depressive disorders).[11] Response to treatment was about twice as likely in the antidepressant group (RR versus placebo 1.9, 95% CI 1.6 to 2.3; NNT 4, 95% CI 3 to 5). **Tricyclic antidepressants (TCAs) versus SSRIs:** We found three systematic reviews comparing SSRIs with TCAs.[12–14] These found no significant difference in effectiveness overall. SSRIs seem to be slightly more acceptable overall as measured by the number of people who withdrew from clinical trials (RR 0.88, 95% CI 0.83 to 0.93; NNT 26).[12] The third systematic review (search date 1998, 28 RCTs, 5940 people) compared the efficacy in primary care of newer antidepressants versus placebo and versus older antidepressants.[14] The average response rate was 63% for newer agents, 35% for placebo, and 60% for TCAs (RR for SSRIs compared with placebo 1.6, 95% CI 1.2 to 2.1). One small RCT (152 people) compared adherence on dothiepin with fluoxetine over 12 weeks and found no significant difference between the drugs. However, the study was probably underpowered.[15] **Monoamine oxidase inhibitors (MAOIs) versus TCAs:** We found one systematic review (search date not given, 55 RCTs comparing MAOIs versus TCAs in several subgroups of people with depression).[16] It found that MAOIs were less effective in people with severe depressive disorders but may be more effective in atypical depressive disorders (depressive disorders with reversed biological features—for example, increased sleep, increased appetite, mood reactivity, and rejection sensitivity). **Older adults:** We identified one systematic review (search date 1998, 40 RCTs of pharmacological and psychological treatments of depression in people older than 55 years), in an outpatient or community setting. Of the trials, 26 were of pharmacological treatments and 21 of these were placebo controlled. People were recruited mainly from outpatient clinics. There was significant heterogeneity in the study results (P = 0.03). Nine heterocyclic drug studies had a mean difference in Hamilton Depression Rating scores after treatment of –5.78 (95% CI –8.31 to –3.25). Significant benefits were also found for fluoxetine, trazodone, and phenelzine. Of the 17 drug versus drug comparisons (mainly involving heterocyclic drugs), none showed significant benefit above the others.[17] **In people with depression plus a physical illness versus placebo:** One systematic review (search date 1998, 18 RCTs, n = 838) found that antidepressants were more effective than placebo in people with depression and a physical illness (NNT 4, 95% CI 3 to 7). People allocated to antidepressants were more likely to withdraw from the study than those on placebo (NNH 10, 95% CI 5 to 43).[18]

Harms:

Common adverse events: One systematic review of RCTs (search date 1996) compared TCAs versus SSRIs in people with all severities of depression (see table 1, p 42).[19] There may also be differences between SSRIs. One large cohort study of people receiving four different SSRIs (fluvoxamine [n = 10 983], fluoxetine [n = 12 692], sertraline [n = 12 734], and paroxetine [n = 13 741]) in British primary care found that reports of common adverse events (nausea/vomiting, malaise/lassitude, dizziness, and headache/migraine) varied between SSRIs (fluvoxamine 78 per 1000 participant months; fluoxetine 23 per 1000 participant months; RR versus fluvoxamine 0.29, 95% CI 0.27 to 0.32; paroxetine 28 per 1000 participant months, RR 0.35, 95% CI 0.33 to 0.37; sertraline 21 per 1000 participant months, RR 0.26, 95% CI 0.25 to 0.28).[20] Only 52% of people responded to the questionnaire, although this response rate was similar for all four drugs. A study of spontaneous reports to the UK Committee on Safety of Medicines found no difference in safety profiles between the same four SSRIs.[21] **Suicide:** One systematic review (which included trials completed by December 1989) pooled data from 17 double blind RCTs in people with depressive disorder comparing fluoxetine (n = 1765) versus a TCA (n = 731) or placebo (n = 569).[22] There was no significant difference in the rate of suicidal acts between the groups (fluoxetine 0.3%, placebo 0.2%, TCAs 0.4%), whereas development of suicidal ideation was less frequent in the fluoxetine group (1.2% fluoxetine *v* 2.6% placebo, P = 0.042, and *v* 3.6% TCAs, P = 0.001). One historical cohort study followed 172 598 people who had at least one prescription for one of 10 antidepressants during the study period in general practice in the UK. The risk of suicide was higher in people who received fluoxetine (19 per 10 000 person years, 95% CI 9 to 34) than those receiving dothiepin (RR of suicide *v* dothiepin 2.1, 95% CI 1.1 to 4.1).[23] In a nested case controlled subanalysis in people with no history of suicidal behaviour or previous antidepressant prescription, the risk remained the same, although the confidence interval broadened to make the result indeterminate (RR 2.1, 95% CI 0.6 to 7.9). Although the apparent association may be due to residual confounding, there remains uncertainty about the possible association between fluoxetine and suicide. However, any absolute increase in risk is unlikely to be large. **Withdrawal effects:** We found one RCT comparing abrupt discontinuation of fluoxetine (n = 96) versus continued treatment (n = 299) in people who had been taking the drug for 12 weeks. Abrupt discontinuation was associated with increased dizziness (7% *v* 1%), dysmenorrhoea (3% *v* 0%), rhinitis (10% *v* 3%), and somnolence (4% *v* 0%). However, there was a high drop out rate in this study because of return of symptoms of depression (39%), so these may be underestimates of the true rate of withdrawal symptoms.[24] The rate of spontaneous reports of suspected withdrawal reactions per million defined daily doses to the World Health Organization Collaborating Centre for International Drug Monitoring between 1987 and 1995 was higher for paroxetine than for sertraline and fluoxetine.[25] The most common withdrawal effects were dizziness, nausea, paraesthesia, headache, and vertigo. **Older adults:** We found no specific evidence on adverse effects in older adults. **During pregnancy:** One systematic review of the risks of fetal harm of antidepressants in pregnancy found four small prospective studies published since 1993.[26] No evidence of increased risk was found, although the chances of adverse effects with a low incidence cannot be excluded. Decreased birth weights of infants exposed to fluoxetine in the third trimester were identified in one study and direct drug effects and withdrawal syndromes were identified in some neonates.

Comment: A systematic review is under way to examine the efficacy of antidepressants in older people, including data on adverse effects.[17] Metabolic and physical changes with age mean that older people may be more prone to adverse effects such as falls. As older people take more medications, they are at more risk of drug interactions. Suicide is a risk in elderly people.

OPTION CARE PATHWAYS

We found limited evidence that effectiveness of drug treatment may be improved by collaborative working between primary care clinicians and psychiatrists, or by intensive patient education.

Benefits: We found no systematic review. We found four RCTs.[27–30] The first in 217 people with mild to moderate depressive disorders in primary care in the USA found that, compared with standard treatment, outcomes were improved by collaborative working between primary care physician and psychiatrist, and by intensive patient education. Clinical outcomes were improved only in the subgroup of people with major depressive disorder (n = 91; AR of clinical response of > 50% reduction on symptom checklist: 74% *v* 44% with standard treatment; NNT 4, 95% CI 3 to 10).[27] The second (613 people) in a Health Maintenance Organization (HMO) in Seattle compared usual care, feedback (in which doctors received a detailed report on each person at 8 and 16 weeks following randomisation), or feedback plus care management (in which the care manager assessed people with depression by telephone at 8 and 16 weeks, doctors received a detailed report, and care managers facilitated the follow up). The care management group were more likely than those treated with usual care to have a clinically significant reduction in depressive symptoms 6 months after randomisation (estimated event rates 40% of the control group *v* 56% of the care management group OR 2.22, 95% CI 1.31 to 3.75; NNT 7).[28] The third RCT (1356 people) in 46 primary care clinics in US HMOs compared a multifaceted quality improvement programme with usual care (including mailed practice guidelines). People in the intervention group improved on continuous rating scales. Among people initially employed, 89.7% of the intervention group worked at 12 months compared with 84.7% of the control group ($P = 0.05$). For people initially not working, there was no difference in employment rates between intervention and control groups at 12 months (17% *v* 18%).[29] The fourth, a cluster randomised RCT in UK primary care, compared the effects of a clinical practice guideline and practice based education with usual care and found that the intervention did not improve either detection or outcome of depression.[30]

Harms: None reported.

Comment: None.

OPTION ST JOHN'S WORT (*HYPERICUM PERFORATUM*)

One systematic review of RCTs has found that St John's Wort (*Hypericum perforatum*) is more effective than placebo in mild to moderate depressive disorders and as effective as prescription antidepressant drugs. However, these findings have yet to be repeated in fully representative groups of people using standardised preparations.

Benefits: We found one systematic review (updated in 1998, 27 RCTs, 2291 people with mild to moderate depression).[31] Of these trials, 17 were placebo controlled (1168 participants). Ten trials (1123 participants) compared hypericum (8 trials used single preparations, 2 used combinations of hypericum and valeriana) versus other antidepressant or sedative drugs. Hypericum preparations were associated with significant clinical improvement compared with placebo (RR 2.47, 95% CI 1.69 to 3.61) but not compared with standard antidepressants (single preparations RR 1.01, 95% CI 0.87 to 1.16, combinations RR 1.52, 95% CI 0.78 to 2.94).

Harms: We found two systematic reviews (one cited above[31] and one other, search date 1997[32]). The review cited above found that adverse events were poorly reported in the trials. They were reported by 26% of people on hypericum compared with 45% of people on standard antidepressants (RR 0.57, 95% CI 0.47 to 0.69) and 15% on combinations of hypericum and valeriana compared with 27% on amitriptyline or desipramine (RR 0.49, 95% CI 0.23 to 1.04).[31] The second systematic review included RCTs and observational post-marketing surveillance studies of hypericum.[32] The commonest adverse effects of hypericum in the included trials were gastrointestinal symptoms, dizziness/confusion, tiredness/sedation, and dry mouth, although all occurred less frequently than on conventional drugs. Findings from observational studies were consistent with these findings. Photosensitivity is theoretically possible; however only two cases have been reported. Allergic skin reactions seem uncommon.

Comment: The evidence cited above must be interpreted cautiously for the following reasons: (1) it is unclear how closely participants in these trials match people in clinical practice; and (2) the preparations and doses of hypericum and types and doses of standard antidepressants varied. More studies are needed on clearly defined, clinically representative people using standardised preparations. Interactions with other drugs are possible and should be considered.

OPTION ELECTROCONVULSIVE THERAPY

One systematic review of RCTs has found that electroconvulsive therapy (ECT) is effective in the acute treatment of depressive illness.

Benefits: We found two systematic reviews. The first (search date not given) included six RCTs and a total of 205 people with depressive disorder that compared ECT versus simulated ECT (in which people received everything but electric stimulation).[33] People treated with real ECT were more likely to respond to treatment (pooled OR 3.7, 95% CI 2.1 to 6.5; NNT 3, 95% CI 2 to 5, calculated from data in the article). The more recent systematic review (search date 1998) included 11 additional RCTs published between 1987 and 1998, but it did not undertake quantitative analysis.[34]

Harms: We found no adequate systematic review of possible adverse cognitive effects of ECT. However, people often complain of memory impairment after ECT. One of the main difficulties in studying this is that depressive disorders also lead to cognitive impairments that usually improve during the course of treatment. For this reason most of the many small studies in this area find an average improvement in people treated with ECT. This does not rule out the possibility of more subtle, subjective memory impairment secondary to ECT. Adverse memory effects would probably vary according to the dose and electrode used.

Comment: The first review cited above[26] did not include several recent RCTs comparing real versus simulated ECT.[35–39] However, the results of these trials are consistent with the review's findings. A further systematic review is in progress.[40] As ECT may be unacceptable to some people and because it is a short term treatment, there is a consensus that it should normally be reserved for people who cannot tolerate or have not responded to drug treatment, although it may be useful when a rapid response is required.

OPTION SPECIFIC PSYCHOLOGICAL TREATMENTS

Younger adults: One systematic review of RCTs has found that cognitive therapy (see glossary, p 39) is effective, and may be more effective than drug treatment in people with mild to moderate depression. Weaker evidence from RCTs suggests that interpersonal psychotherapy, problem solving therapy and brief, non-directive counselling (see glossary, p 39) may be as effective as drug treatment in mild to moderate depression. We found limited evidence on the relative efficacy of drug and non-drug treatment in severe depression. Older adults: One systematic review of RCTs has found that rational psychological treatments (such as cognitive therapy or cognitive behaviour therapy) are effective for older people with mild to moderate depression. However, people receiving these treatments

improved no more than controls who received similar but non-specific attention. This review was based on a small number of studies, the populations varied (although most were community samples), and many of the studies were short term.

Benefits: **Younger adults:** The evidence comparing psychological treatments versus drug or no treatment is summarised in table 2, p 43.[41–43] **Older adults:** We identified one systematic review of 40 controlled trials of pharmacological and psychological treatments in people over the age of 55 in an outpatient or community setting.[44] The review found four comparisons in older adults of psychological treatments (such as psychotherapy) versus untreated controls. None of the trials found a significant difference between treatment and no treatment, measured on the Hamilton Depression Rating Scale. The review also identified six comparisons of different psychological treatments. None found significant differences in effectiveness. Five of six comparisons of "rational" treatments (such as cognitive therapy or cognitive behaviour therapy) versus no treatment in older adults found significant benefit with treatment. Combined, the rational treatments performed significantly better than no treatment, with a mean difference in the Hamilton Depression Rating score of –7.25 (95% CI, –10.1 to –4.4). However, neither of the two rational treatments performed significantly better than non-specific attention.

Harms: See table 2, p 43.

Comment: Large RCTs are needed in more representative people in a range of clinical settings, including primary care. Because of varying exclusion criteria, the generaliseability of the studies is questionable (see table 2, p 43). Other factors to be considered when psychological treatments are compared with drug treatment include whether serum concentrations of drugs reach therapeutic concentrations, whether changes in medication are allowed (reflecting standard clinical practice), and whether studies reflect the natural course of depressive disorders.

OPTION SPECIFIC PSYCHOLOGICAL TREATMENTS PLUS DRUG TREATMENT

We found evidence from RCTs suggesting that, in severe depression, the addition of drug treatment to interpersonal or cognitive therapy is more effective than either psychological therapy alone. No such effect was observed in mild to moderate depression.

Benefits: We found no systematic review. A non-systematic meta-analysis of six RCTs (595 people) found no advantage in combining drug and specific psychological treatments in mild to moderate depressive disorders, but that in more severe depressive disorders, combining drug and interpersonal therapy or cognitive therapy was more effective than interpersonal therapy or cognitive therapy alone.[45] One recent RCT compared nefazodone or cognitive behavioural–analysis psychotherapy alone with combination treatment in 681 adults with chronic depressive disorder.[46] At 12 weeks, the combined treatment improved the rate of clinical response (at least

50% reduction on the Hamilton Depression Rating Scale and a score of 15 or less, combined therapy *v* both single interventions, NNT 5, 95% CI 3 to 6).

Harms: We found no evidence of adverse effects.

Comment: A systematic review is needed to address this question.

OPTION EXERCISE

RCTs have found that exercise, alone or combined with other treatments, improves mild to moderate depression.

Benefits: We found one systematic review (published in 1990, search date not given), which examined exercise in depressive disorders. However, it was difficult to interpret because it included non-randomised studies and did not clearly describe participants.[47] One small RCT (156 people) compared aerobic exercise, sertraline hydrochloride (an SSRI), and combined treatment for 16 weeks. It found that all groups improved on continuous rating scales, but there was no significant difference in overall improvement between treatments.[48]

Harms: None reported.

Comment: None.

OPTION BIBLIOTHERAPY

We found limited evidence from a systematic review of RCTs that bibliotherapy (see glossary, p 39) may reduce mild depressive symptoms.

Benefits: We found one systematic review (published in 1997). It identified six small short term RCTs of bibliotherapy in 273 participants recruited by advertisement through the media and probably only mildly ill.[49] The mean effect size of bibliotherapy was 0.82 (95% CI 0.50 to 1.15). This means that 79% of control people had a worse outcome than the average member of the group receiving bibliotherapy.

Harms: None reported.

Comment: Further studies are needed in clinically representative groups.

OPTION BEFRIENDING

Limited evidence from one small RCT found that befriending reduced symptoms of depression.

Benefits: We found one small RCT (86 people) of befriending (see glossary, p 39) of women with chronic depression in London. Initial identification was by postal screening of women registered with but not attending primary care.[50] It found that the befriended group were more likely to experience remission of symptoms at 13 months (65% with befriending *v* 39% with control; $P < 0.05$; NNT 4, 95% CI 2 to 18).

Harms: None recorded.

Comment: Less than half of the women screened were interested in befriending as a treatment option.

QUESTION What are the effects of continuation and maintenance treatment with antidepressant drugs?

RCTs have found that continuation treatment (see glossary, p 39) with antidepressant drugs for 4–6 months after recovery reduces risk of relapse.

Benefits: **Continuation treatment:** We found one systematic review (published in 1991, 6 RCTs, 312 people).[51] Continuation of antidepressant medication for 4–6 months after acute treatment reduced the relapse rate by nearly half (RR 0.6, 95% CI 0.4 to 0.7). Several more recent RCTs confirm this reduction in risk of early relapse with continuing antidepressant treatment for 6–12 months after acute treatment. **Maintenance treatment:** We found no adequate systematic review, but several RCTs have found that maintenance treatment reduced the relapse rate compared with placebo in recurrent depressive disorder. However, they all have problems with their methods (e.g. high withdrawal rates[52]), and will be considered for the next issue of *Clinical Evidence*. **Older adults:** We found one RCT that compared dothiepin versus placebo in 69 older people who had recovered sufficiently and consented to enter a 2 year trial of continuation treatment.[53] Dothiepin reduced the risk of relapse by 55% (RR 0.45, 95% CI 0.22 to 0.96).

Harms: Adverse effects seem to be similar to those reported in trials of acute treatment.

Comment: A systematic review is in progress.[54]

QUESTION Which treatments are most effective at improving long term outcome?

We found no evidence of a difference between treatments in terms of long term benefits. We found limited evidence that cognitive therapy may be an alternative to drug maintenance therapy in preventing relapse.

Benefits: We found one systematic review (published in 1998, search date not given), which identified eight small RCTs examining long term (at least 1 year) recovery or relapse rates after treatment had stopped. The trials compared cognitive therapy versus antidepressants in people with mainly mild to moderate depressive disorders.[41] Overall, 30% of people[16] treated with cognitive therapy relapsed compared with 60% of those treated with antidepressants. However, the number of people in these trials was too small for this trend to be significant. We found one small additional RCT (40 people) comparing cognitive therapy with normal clinical management for residual depressive symptoms in people who had responded to antidepressants. It also found that at 2 years fewer people relapsed with cognitive therapy than with antidepressants.[55]

Harms: See harms of prescription antidepressant drugs, p 32 and see table 2, p 43.

Comment: The review did not present data on the proportion of people who recovered and remained well in the long term. The largest RCT found that only a fifth of participants remained well over 18 months' follow up, and that there were no significant differences between interpersonal psychotherapy, cognitive therapy, or drug treatment.[43] It is possible that different people respond to different treatments. Further large scale comparative studies are needed of the long term effectiveness of treatments in people with all severities of depressive disorders.

GLOSSARY

Bibliotherapy Consists of advising people to read written material such as *Feeling good: the new mood therapy* by David Burns (New York: New American Library 1980).

Brief, non-directive counselling Aims to help people to express feelings and clarify thoughts and difficulties; therapist suggests alternative understandings and does not give direct advice but tries to encourage people to solve their own problems.

Cognitive therapy Brief (20 sessions over 12–16 weeks) structured treatment aimed at changing the dysfunctional beliefs and negative automatic thoughts that characterise depressive disorders. It requires a high level of training in the therapist.[56]

Continuation treatment Continuation of treatment after successful resolution of a depressive episode to prevent relapse.

Interpersonal psychotherapy Standardised form of brief psychotherapy (usually 12–16 weekly sessions) primarily intended for outpatients with unipolar non-psychotic depressive disorders. It focuses on improving the patient's interpersonal functioning and identifying the problems associated with the onset of the depressive episode.[57]

Maintenance treatment Long term treatment of recurrent depressive disorder to prevent the recurrence of further depressive episodes.

Problem solving Consists of three stages: (1) identifying the main problems for the patient; (2) generating solutions; (3) trying out the solutions. Potentially briefer and simpler than cognitive therapy and may be feasible in primary care.[43]

Befriending Consists of a befriender meeting the patient to talk and socialise for at least 1 hour per week, acting as a friend.

Substantive changes since last issue of Clinical Evidence

TCAs versus SSRIs Two systematic reviews;[12,13] one new systematic review comparing the efficacy in primary care of newer antidepressants with placebo and older antidepressants;[14] and one new RCT;[15] conclusions unchanged.

People with depression plus a physical illness One new systematic review found that antidepressants were more effective than placebo.[18]

Pregnancy One new systematic review of the risks of fetal harm of antidepressants in pregnancy.[26] No evidence of increased risk for intrauterine death or major birth defects was reported. The development of children whose mothers took TCAs or fluoxetine during gestation did not differ from controls. Decreased birth weights of infants exposed to fluoxetine in the third trimester were identified in one study and direct drug effects and withdrawal syndromes were identified in some neonates.

Care pathways Three new RCTs; conclusions unchanged.[28–30]

Electroconvulsive therapy Two new RCTs; conclusions unchanged.[38,39]

Specific psychological treatments plus drug treatment One recent RCT found combination therapy was more effective than nefazodone or cognitive behavioural–analysis psychotherapy alone.[46]

Exercise One recent RCT; conclusion unchanged.[48]

Improving long term outcome One new RCT found limited evidence that cognitive therapy may be an alternative to drug maintenance therapy in preventing relapse.[55]

REFERENCES

1. Rosenstein, Leslie D. Differential diagnosis of the major progressive dementias and depression in middle and late adulthood: a summary of the literature of the early 1990s. *Neuropsychol Rev* 1998;8:109–167.
2. Katon W, Schulberg H. Epidemiology of depression in primary care. *Gen Hosp Psychiatry* 1992:14: 237–247.
3. Murray CJ, Lopez AD. Regional patterns of disability-free life expectancy and disability–adjusted life expectancy: global burden of disease study. *Lancet* 1997;349:1347–1352.
4. Murray CJ, Lopez AD. Alternative projections of mortality and disability by cause 1990–2020: global burden of disease study. *Lancet* 1997;349: 1498–1504.
5. Beekman ATF, Copeland JRM, Prince MJ. Review of community prevalence of depression in later life. *Br J Psychiatry* 1999;174:307–11.
6. Judd LL, Akiskal HS, Maser JD, et al. A prospective 12 year study of subsyndromal and syndromal depressive symptoms in unipolar major depressive disorders. *Arch Gen Psychiatry* 1988; 55:694–700.
7. American Psychiatric Association. *Diagnostic and statistical manual of mental disorders*, 4th ed. Washington, DC: American Psychiatric Association, 1994.
8. World Health Organization. *The ICD-10 classification of mental and behavioural disorders*. Geneva: World Health Organization, 1992.
9. Cole MG, Bellavance F, Mansour A. Prognosis of depression in elderly community and primary care populations: a systematic review and meta-analysis. *Am J Psychiatry* 1999;156:1182–1189.
10. Joffe R, Sokolov S, Streiner D. Antidepressant treatment of depression: a meta-analysis. *Can J Psychiatry* 1996;41:613–616. Search date not given; primary source Medline 1966 to June 1995.
11. Lima MS, Moncrieff J. A comparison of drugs versus placebo for the treatment of dysthymia: a systematic review. In: Cochrane library, Issue 3, 1998. Oxford: Update Software. Search date 1997; primary sources Biological Abstracts 1984 to 1997; Medline 1966 to January 1997; Psychlit 1974 to January 1997; Embase 1980 to January 1997; Lilacs 1982 to January 1997; Cochrane library; personal communication; conference abstracts; unpublished trials from the pharmaceutical industry; and book chapters on the treatment of depression.
12. Geddes JR, Freemantle N, Mason J, Eccles MP, Boynton J SSRIs versus other antidepressants for depressive disorder. In: The Cochrane Library, Issue 3, 2000. Oxford: Update software. Search date 1999; primary source Medline, Embase, Cochrane Group Register of Controlled Trials, hand searches of reference lists of all located studies, and contact with manufacturers.
13. Anderson IM. Selective serotonin reuptake inhibitors versus tricyclic antidepressants: a meta-analysis of efficacy and tolerability. *J Affect Disord* 2000;58:19–36. Search date 1997; primary sources Medline, and hand searches of reference lists of meta-analyses and reviews.
14. Mulrow CD, Williams JW, Chiqueete E, et al. Efficacy of newer medications for treating depression in primary care patients. *Am Med J* 2000;108:54–64. Search date 1998; primary source Cochrane Depression Anxiety and Neurosis Group Specialised Register of Clinical Trials, hand searches of trials and 46 pertinent meta-analyses and consultation with experts.
15. Thompson C, Peveler RC, Stephenson D, et al. Compliance with antidepressant medication in the treatment of major depressive disorder in primary care: a randomized comparison of fluoxetine and a tricyclic antidepressant. *Am J Psychiatry* 2000; 157:338–343.
16. Thase ME, Trivedi MH, Rush AJ. MAOIs in the contemporary treatment of depression. *Neuropsychopharmacology* 1995;12:185–219. Search date not given; primary sources Medline and Psychological Abstracts 1959–July 1992.
17. Wilson K, Mottram P, Sivanthan A. A review of antidepressant drug trials in the treatment of older depressed people (protocol for a Cochrane Review). In: The Cochrane Library. Issue 4, 1998. Oxford: Update software. Search date June 1998; primary sources Cochrane Depression, Neurosis and Anxiety Review Group; hand searched journals, and reference lists. Review not to be published until 2001.
18. Gill D, Hatcher S. Antidepressants for depression in people with physical illness. In: The Cochrane Library, Issue 3, 2000. Oxford: Update software. Search date 1998; primary sources Medline, Cochrane Library Trials Register, Cochrane Depression and Neurosis Group Trials Register, and hand searches of two journals and reference lists.
19. Trindade E, Menon D. Selective serotonin reuptake inhibitors differ from tricyclic antidepressants in adverse events [abstract]. *Selective serotonin reuptake inhibitors (SSRIs) for major depression. Part I. Evaluation of the clinical literature*. Ottawa: Canadian Coordinating Office for Health Technology Assessment, 1997 August Report 3E. *Evidence-Based Mental Health* 1998;1:50. Search date 1996; primary sources Medline; Embase; PsycINFO; International Pharmaceutical Abstracts; Pascal; Health Planning and Administration; Mental Health Abstracts; Pharmacoeconomics and Outcomes News; Current Contents databases; scanning bibliographies of retrieved articles; hand searching journals; consulting researchers.
20. Mackay FJ, Dunn NR, Wilton LV, et al. A comparison of fluvoxamine, fluoxetine, sertraline and paroxetine examined by observational cohort studies. *Pharmacoepidemiol Drug Safety* 1997;6: 235–246.
21. Price JS, Waller PC, Wood SM, et al. A comparison of the post marketing safety of four selective serotonin reuptake inhibitors including the investigation of symptoms occurring on withdrawal. *Br J Clin Pharmacol* 1996;42:757–763.
22. Beasley CM Jr, Dornseif BE, Bosomworth JC, et al. Fluoxetine and suicide: a meta-analysis of controlled trials of treatment for depression. *BMJ*

1991;303:685–692. Search date not given; but included trials that had been completed/analysed by December 1989; primary sources not given in detail but based on clinical report form data from trials and data from the Drug Experience Network Database.

23. Jick SS, Dean AD, Jick H. Antidepressants and suicide. *BMJ* 1995;310:215–218.
24. Zajecka J, Fawcett J, Amsterdam J, et al. Safety of abrupt discontinuation of fluoxetine: a randomised, placebo controlled study. *J Clin Psychopharmacol* 1998;18:193–197.
25. Stahl MM, Lindquist M, Pettersson M, et al. Withdrawal reactions with selective serotonin reuptake inhibitors as reported to the WHO system. *Eur J Clin Pharmacol* 1997;53:163–169.
26. Wisner KL, Gelenberg AJ, Leonard H, et al. Pharmacologic treatment of depression during pregnancy. *JAMA* 1999;282:1264–1269. Search date 1999; primary sources Medline, Healthstar, hand searches of bibliographies of review articles, and discussions with investigators in the field.
27. Katon W, Von Korff M, Lin E, et al. Collaborative management to achieve treatment guidelines: impact on depression in primary care. *JAMA* 1995;273:1026–1031.
28. Simon GE, Vonkorff M, Rutter C, et al. Randomised trial of monitoring, feedback, and management of care by telephone to improve treatment of depression in primary care. *BMJ* 2000;320:550–554.
29. Wells KB, Sherbourne C, Schoenbaum M, et al. Impact of disseminating quality improvement programs for depression in managed primary care: a randomized controlled trial. *JAMA* 2000;283: 212–220.
30. Thompson C, Kinmonth AL, Stevens L, et al. Effects of a clinical-practice guideline and practice-based education on detection and outcome of depression in primary care: Hampshire Depression Project randomised controlled trial. *Lancet* 2000;355:185–191.
31. Linde K, Mulrow CD. St John's Wort for depression. In: The Cochrane Library. Issue 4, 1998. Oxford: Update software. Search date 1998; primary sources Medline 1983 to 1997; Embase 1989 to 1997; PsychLit 1987 to 1997; Psychindex 1987 to 1997; specialised databases: Cochrane Complementary Medicine Field, Cochrane Depression and Neurosis CRG, Phytodok; bibliographies of pertinent articles; manufacturers and researchers.
32. Ernst E, Rand JI, Barnes J, et al. Adverse effects profile of the herbal antidepressant St John Wort (*Hypericum perforatum L*) *Eur J Clin Pharmacol* 1998;54:589–594. Search date September 1997; primary sources AMED 1985 to September 1997; Cochrane Library 1997 Issue 2; Embase 1980 to September 1997, Medline 1996 to September 1997; handsearched reference lists; contacted WHO Collaborating Centre for International Drug Monitoring; UK Committee on Safety of Medicines and German Bundesinstitut f r Arzneimittel und Medizinproducte plus 12 German manufacturers of hypericum products.
33. Janicak PG, Davis JM, Gibbons RD, et al. Efficacy of ECT: a meta-analysis. *Am J Psychiatry* 1985; 142:297–302. Search date not given; primary source Medline.
34. Wijeratne GS, Halliday GS, Lyndon RW. The present status of electroconvulsive therapy: a systematic review. *Med J Austr* 1999;171:250–254. Search date 1998; primary source Medline 1987 to 1998.
35. Johnstone EC, Deakin JF, Lawler P, et al. The Northwick Park electroconvulsive therapy trial. *Lancet* 1980;1:1317–1320.
36. Brandon S, Cowley P, McDonald C, et al. Electroconvulsive therapy: results in depressive illness from the Leicestershire trial. *BMJ* 1984; 288:22–25.
37. Gregory S, Shawcross CR, Gill D. The Nottingham ECT study. A double-blind comparison of bilateral, unilateral and simulated ECT in depressive illness. *Br J Psychiatry* 1985;146:520–524.
38. Vaughan McCall W, Reboussin DM, Weiner RD, et al Titrated moderately suprathreshold vs fixed high-dose right unilateral electroconvulsive therapy. *Arch Gen Psychiatry* 2000;57:438–444 .
39. Sackeim HA, Prudic J, Devanand DP, et al. A prospective, randomized, double-blind comparison of bilateral and right unilateral electroconvulsive therapy at different stimulus intensities. *Arch Gen Psychiatry* 2000;57:425–434.
40. Scott AIF, Doris AB. Electroconvulsive therapy for depression (protocol). In: The Cochrane Library. Issue 4, 1998. Oxford: Update software.
41. Gloaguen V, Cottraux J, Cucherat M, et al. A meta-analysis of the effects of cognitive therapy in depressed patients 1998. *J Affect Disord* 1998; 49:59–72. Search date not given; primary sources Medline 1966 to December 1996; Embase 1966 to December 1996; references in books and papers; previous reviews and meta-analyses; abstracts from congress presentations; preprints sent by authors.
42. Elkin I, Shea MT, Watkins JT, et al. National Institute of Mental Health treatment of depression collaborative research program: general effectiveness of treatments. *Arch Gen Psychiatry* 1989;46:971–982.
43. Mynors-Wallis LM, Gath DH, Lloyd-Thomas, AR, et al. Randomised controlled trial comparing problem solving treatment with amitriptyline and placebo for major depression in primary care. *BMJ* 1995; 310:441–445.
44. Churchill R, Dewey M, Gretton V, et al. Should general practitioners refer patients with major depression to counsellors? A review of current published evidence. *Br J Gen Pract* 1999;49: 738–743.
45. Thase ME, Greenhouse JB, Frank E, et al. Treatment of major depression with psychotherapy or psychotherapy—pharmacotherapy combinations. *Arch Gen Psychiatry* 1997;54: 1009–1015. Pooled results of six research protocols conducted 1982 to 1992 at the Mental Health Clinical Research Center, University of Pittsburgh School of Medicine.
46. Keller MB, McCullough JP, Klein DN, et al. A comparison of nefazodone, the cognitive behavioral-analysis system of psychotherapy, and their combination for the treatment of chronic depression. *N Engl J Med* 2000;342:1462–1470.
47. North TC, McCullagh P, Tran ZV. Effect of exercise on depression. *Exerc Sport Sci Rev* 1990;18:379–415. Search date not given; primary sources dissertation abstracts online, ERIC, PsychInfo, Medline, books, abstracts from meetings to June 1989.
48. Blumenthal JA, Babyak MA, Moore KA, et al. Effects of exercise training on older patients with major depression. *Arch Intern Med* 1999;159: 2349–2356.
49. Cuijpers P. Bibliotherapy in unipolar depression: a meta-analysis. *J Behav Ther Exp Psychiatry* 1997; 28:139–147. Search date not given; primary sources Psychlit; Psychinfo; Medline.
50. Harris T, Brown GW, Robinson R. Befriending as an intervention for chronic depression among women in an inner city: Randomised controlled trial. *Br J Psychiatry* 1999;174:219–224.
51. Loonen AJ, Peer PG, Zwanikken GJ. Continuation and maintenance therapy with antidepressive

agents: meta-analysis of research. *Pharm Week Sci* 1991;13:167–175. Search date not given; primary sources references of textbooks and review articles; Medline 1977 to 1988; Embase 1977 to 1988; review of reference lists of primary studies.

52. Keller MB, Kocsis JH, Thase ME, et al. Maintenance phase efficacy of sertraline for chronic depression: a randomized controlled trial. *JAMA* 1998;280:1665–1672.
53. Old age depression interest group. How long should the elderly take antidepressants? A double-blind placebo-controlled study of continuation/prophylaxis therapy with dothiepin. *Br J Psychiatry* 1993;162:175–182.
54. Carney S, Geddes J, Davies D, Furukawa T, Kupfer D, Goodwin G. Duration of treatment with antidepressants in depressive disorder (protocol). In: The Cochrane Library, Issue 3 2000. Oxford: Update software.
55. Fava GA, Rafanelli C, Grandi S, et al. Prevention of recurrent depression with cognitive behavioral therapy: preliminary findings. *Arch Gen Psychiatry* 1998;55:816–820.
56. Haaga DAF, Beck AT. Cognitive therapy. In: Paykel ES, ed. *Handbook of affective disorders.* Edinburgh: Churchill Livingstone, 1992:511–523.
57. Klerman GL, Weissman H. Interpersonal psychotherapy. In: Paykel ES, ed. *Handbook of affective disorders.* Edinburgh: Churchill Livingstone, 1992:501–510.

John Geddes
Senior Clinical Research Fellow/Honorary Consultant Psychiatrist
University of Oxford
Oxford
UK

Rob Butler
Lecturer in Old Age Psychiatry

James Warner
Senior Lecturer/Consultant in Old Age Psychiatry

Imperial College School of Medicine
London
UK

Competing interests: None declared.

TABLE 1 Adverse events (% of patients) with selective serotonin reuptake inhibitors (SSRIs) versus tricyclic antidepressants (TCAs) (see text, p 32).[20]

Adverse effects	SSRIs event rates (%)	TCAs event rates (%)
Dry mouth	21	55
Constipation	10	22
Dizziness	13	23
Nausea	22	12
Diarrhoea	13	5
Anxiety	13	7
Agitation	14	8
Insomnia	12	7
Nervousness	15	11
Headache	17	14

TABLE 2 Effects of specific psychological treatments for depressive disorders (see text, p 36).

Intervention	Evidence	Benefits	Harms/disadvantages
Cognitive therapy	One systematic review identified 48 RCTs of psychological therapies (n = 2765 people, mainly outpatients in secondary care therefore probably with mild to moderate depression; people with psychotic or bipolar symptoms were excluded). Twenty RCTs compared cognitive therapy with waiting list or placebo and 17 compared it with drug treatment.[33]	79% of people in the placebo control group were more symptomatic than the average person treated with cognitive therapy (effect size 0.82, 95% CI 0.81 to 0.83).[32] 65% of people treated with cognitive therapy were less symptomatic than the average person treated with antidepressant drugs (effect size –0.38, 95% CI –0.39 to –0.37).[32]	No harms reported. Requires extensive training. Limited availability. RCTs in primary care suggest limited acceptability to some people.
Interpersonal psychotherapy	No systematic reviews. One large RCT, including people with mild to moderate depressive disorders, compared interpersonal psychotherapy versus drug treatment, cognitive therapy, or placebo plus clinical management of 16 weeks' duration.[33]	Recovery rates were: placebo-clinical management (21%); interpersonal psychotherapy (43%, NNT 5, 95% CI 3 to 19), imipramine (42%, NNT 5, 95% CI 3 to 22).[33]	No harms reported. Requires extensive training. Limited availability.
Problem solving therapy	No systematic reviews. Several small RCTs comparing problem solving versus drug treatment in primary care in people with mild depressive disorders.[35]	Problem solving was as effective as drug treatment.	No harms reported. Requires some training. Limited availability.
Non-directive counselling	One systematic review identified five RCTs comparing counselling with routine GP managemenet in UK primary care.[35] The RCTs included people with depressive disorders. There is also a protocol registered with the Cochrane database.[36]	No quantitative results provided in review. No consistent improvement in main outcomes, although studies report higher levels of satisfaction with treatment in counselling.	No harms reported. Requires some training. Limited availability.

Depression in children and adolescents

Philip Hazell

QUESTIONS

INTERVENTIONS

Covered elsewhere in this issue
See depressive disorders, p 28.

See glossary, p 48

Key Messages

- One systematic review has found evidence of no benefit from tricyclic antidepressants in prepubertal children, and no clear benefit in adolescents. Fluoxetine may be of some benefit in child and adolescent depression, but more research is needed. We found no evidence to support the use of other serotonin reuptake inhibitor drugs. We found equivocal evidence to support the use of the reversible monoamine oxidase inhibitor moclobemide. We found no evidence supporting the use of non-reversible monoamine oxidase inhibitors. Preliminary data do not support the use of the selective noradrenergic reuptake inhibitor venlafaxine, nor the mood stabiliser lithium.
- We found insufficient evidence on the effects of St John's Wort *(Hypericum perforatum)* and electroconvulsive therapy in children and adolescents with depression.
- One systematic review of RCTs has found cognitive behavioural therapy to be superior to non-specific supportive therapies for mild to moderate depression in children and adolescents. Two RCTs of interpersonal therapy also suggested benefit compared with no treatment. We found insufficient evidence to conclude that family therapy, or group treatments other than cognitive behavioural therapy, are effective treatments for depression in children and adolescents.
- We found no systematic reviews or RCTs looking at long term outcomes for psychological or pharmacological treatments.

DEFINITION See depressive disorders, p 28. Compared with adult depression, depression in children and adolescents may have a more insidious onset, may be characterised more by irritability than sadness, and occurs more often in association with other conditions such as anxiety, conduct disorder, hyperkinesis, and learning problems.[1]

INCIDENCE/ PREVALENCE Estimates of prevalence of depression among children and adolescents in the community range from 1.7% to 5.9%.[2,3] Prevalence tends to increase with age, with a sharp rise around onset of puberty. Pre-adolescent boys and girls are equally affected by the condition, but depression is seen more frequently among adolescent girls than boys.[4]

AETIOLOGY/ RISK FACTORS Causes are uncertain, including childhood events and current psychosocial adversity.

PROGNOSIS See prognosis under depressive disorders, p 28. In children and adolescents, the recurrence rate of depressive episodes first occurring in childhood or adolescence is 70% by 5 years, which is similar to the recurrence rate in adults.[5] Young people experiencing a moderate to severe depressive episode may be more likely than adults to have a manic episode within the next few years.[4] Trials of treatment for child and adolescent depression have found high rates of spontaneous remission (as much as two thirds of people in some inpatient studies).

AIMS To improve mood, social and occupational functioning, and quality of life; to reduce morbidity and mortality; to prevent recurrence of depressive disorder; and to minimise adverse effects of treatment.

OUTCOMES See depressive disorders, p 28. In children and adolescents, there are developmentally specific continuous measures such as the Children's Depression Rating Scale and the Children's Depression Inventory. Categorical outcomes are sometimes expressed as patients no longer meeting DSM criteria for depression on a structured psychiatric interview such as the Kiddie-SADS.

METHODS *Clinical Evidence* update search and appraisal May 2000. Subsequent author search for systematic reviews in The Cochrane Library 2000, Issue 3.

QUESTION What are the effects of treatments?

OPTION PRESCRIPTION ANTIDEPRESSANT DRUGS

One systematic review has found no evidence of benefit from tricyclic antidepressants in prepubertal children, and no clear benefit in adolescents. We have found limited evidence that fluoxetine may be of some benefit for child and adolescent depression. We found no evidence about other serotonin reuptake inhibitor drugs. We found little high quality evidence regarding moclobemide. We found no evidence on the effectiveness of non-reversible monoamine oxidase inhibitors. We have found no evidence that venlafaxine or lithium are beneficial, although the power of the trials was too low to rule out a clinically important difference.

Benefits: **Tricyclic antidepressants:** We found one systematic review (search date 1997, 14 RCTs)[6] and one subsequent RCT.[7] The systematic review found no significant reduction in non-response with the active drug versus placebo (n = 273; OR 0.83, 95% CI 0.48 to 1.42). Analyses for children (2 trials) and adolescents (5 trials) also found no significant benefit of treatment, (children RR of failure to recover 0.9, 95% CI 0.7 to 1.2; adolescents RR of failure to recover 0.9, 95% CI 0.7 to 1.3). However, using the weighted mean difference, trials found a modest but significant difference in adolescents (WMD in depression checklist scores –2.3, 95% CI –3.3 to –1.4) but not in children. Inclusion of the subsequent RCT (meta-analysis personal communication from the author) produced little changes in the estimate of effectiveness but narrowed the 95% confidence intervals.[7] **Pulsed intravenous clomipramine:** We found no systematic review. One small RCT including 16 non-suicidal adolescent outpatients with major depression found that significantly more people responded to intravenous clomipramine 200 mg than to saline.[8] **Monoamine oxidase inhibitors:** We found no systematic review. In one small RCT, 20 adolescents treated with moclobemide showed greater improvement on one clinician rated scale than those treated with placebo, but not on other clinician rated and self report measures.[9] We found no trials of non-reversible monoamine oxidase inhibitors. **Selective serotonin reuptake inhibitors:** We found one systematic review (search date 1998, two RCTs, n = 126).[10] The first RCT in the systematic review (n = 30) found no global benefit. The second RCT (n = 96) found significant benefit on clinician reported global rating and on self reported depressive symptoms, but not on other measures. The systematic review did not pool data from the two RCTs. However, combination of the results for clinician global rating, using a random effects model, found an insignificant pooled odds ratio for non-improvement (0.5, 95% CI 0.22 to 1.12). **Selective noradrenergic reuptake inhibitors:** We found one systematic review (search date 1998, one RCT, n = 33).[10] The one small RCT compared a combination of venlafaxine and psychotherapy with a combination of placebo and psychotherapy. It found no significant difference with regard to improvement. **Lithium:** We found no systematic review. One small placebo controlled RCT compared lithium versus placebo in 30 depressed prepubertal children with a family history of bipolar affective disorder.[11] It found no significant difference of global assessment or of depression scores at follow up.

Harms: See harms of antidepressants under depressive disorders, p 28. One systematic review awaiting publication found that tricyclic antidepressants were more commonly associated with vertigo (OR 8.47, 95% CI 1.40 to 51.0), orthostatic hypotension (OR 4.77, 95% CI 1.11 to 20.5) and dry mouth (OR 5.19, 95% CI 1.15 to 23.5) than placebo (P Hazell et al, personal communication, 2000). It found no significant differences for other adverse effects (tiredness, sleep problems, headache, palpitations, tremor, perspiration, constipation, or problems with micturition). We found single case reports and case series of toxicity and death from tricyclic antidepressants in overdose and therapeutic doses. See harms of antidepressants under depressive disorders, p 28. Of the 17 children randomised to lithium treatment, four were withdrawn because of adverse effects (three had confusion, one had nausea and vomiting).[11]

Comment: Further research is needed to determine long term effects of intravenous clomipramine.

OPTION **ST JOHN'S WORT (*HYPERICUM PERFORATUM*)**

We found no evidence about the effects of St John's Wort (*Hypericum perforatum*) in children and adolescents with depression.

Benefits: We found no systematic review and no RCTs in children or adolescents.

Harms: See harms of St John's Wort under depressive disorders, p 28. We found no evidence about adverse effects in children and adolescents.

Comment: None.

OPTION **ELECTROCONVULSIVE THERAPY**

We found insufficient evidence about the routine use of electroconvulsive therapy in children and adolescents with depression.

Benefits: We found no systematic reviews or RCTs.

Harms: Despite widespread concern about potentially harmful effects of electroconvulsive therapy, especially on memory loss, we found no evidence about harms in children or adolescents.

Comment: None.

OPTION **SPECIFIC PSYCHOLOGICAL TREATMENTS**

One systematic review of RCTs has found cognitive behavioural therapy increases the rate of resolution of the symptoms of depression compared with non-specific supportive therapies for children and adolescents with mild to moderate depression. One RCT of interpersonal therapy found slightly more people recovered than with clinical monitoring alone. A further RCT did not find a significant difference in the recovery rate with interpersonal therapy compared with waiting list control. We found insufficient evidence to conclude that family therapy, or group treatments other than cognitive behavioural therapy, are effective treatments for depression in children and adolescents.

Benefits: **Cognitive behavioural therapy:** See glossary, p 48. We found one systematic review (search date 1997, 6 RCTs, 376 people) of cognitive behavioural therapy compared with "inactive" treatment that ranged from waiting list control to supportive psychotherapy.[12] Cognitive behavioural therapy was associated with increased rate of resolution of symptoms of depression (OR 3.2, 95% CI 1.9 to 5.2; NNT 4, 95% CI 3 to 5) a finding consistent with two non-systematic meta-analytic studies.[13,14] **Interpersonal therapy:** See glossary, p 49. We found no systematic review. We found two RCTs that compared twelve weekly sessions of interpersonal therapy versus clinical monitoring or waiting list control in adolescents with depression. In the first RCT, sessions were augmented by telephone contact. In the first RCT (n = 48) 18 of 24 adolescents receiving treatment interpersonal therapy recovered versus 11 of 24 adolescents receiving clinical monitoring alone (RR 1.64, 95% CI 1.00 to 2.68; ARR 0.29, 95% CI 0.03 to 0.56).[15] In the second RCT (n = 46) 17 of 19 adolescents receiving interpersonal therapy recovered versus 12 of 18 adolescents on the waiting list (RR 1.33, 95% CI 0.94 to 1.93; ARR 0.22, 95% CI –0.03 to +0.49).[16] **Family therapy:** We found no systematic review. One RCT of family therapy versus non-specific supportive therapy did not find a significant difference in remission rates (29% *v* 34%).[17] **Group administered cognitive behavioural therapy:** We found no systematic review. In one RCT group administered cognitive behavioural therapy for adolescents with depression produced a significantly higher remission rate amongst those receiving treatment (67%) compared with those on a waiting list (48%).[18] **Group therapeutic support versus group social skills training:** We found no systematic review. One RCT in 47 adolescents comparing group therapeutic support versus group social skills training found no significant difference in remission rates (50% *v* 40%).[19]

Harms: See harms of specific psychological treatments under depressive disorders, p 28. We found no report of harms specifically for children and adolescents.

Comment: See comment of specific psychological treatments under depressive disorders, p 28.

QUESTION **Which treatments are most effective at improving long term outcome?**

We found no systematic reviews and no RCTs looking at long term outcomes.

Benefits: We found no systematic reviews and no RCTs. We found no trials comparing structured psychotherapy with pharmacotherapy in children and adolescents. We found no trials comparing combined pharmacotherapy and psychotherapy with either treatment alone. We found no trials comparing different psychotherapies.

Harms: See harms of cognitive behavioural therapy, p 47 and harms of prescription antidepressant drugs, p 46.

Comment: See depressive disorders, p 28. We found one prospective cohort study in which adolescents with depression, randomised to cognitive behavioural therapy, systemic behavioural family therapy, or nondirective supportive therapy, were assessed at 3 monthly intervals for the first 12 months and then once again at 24 months. The study found no significant difference between the groups. Of 106 adolescents, 38% experienced sustained recovery, 21% experienced persistent depression, and 41% had a relapsing course.[20]

GLOSSARY

Cognitive behavioural therapy A brief (20 sessions over 12–16 weeks) structured treatment aimed at changing the dysfunctional beliefs and negative automatic thoughts that characterise depressive disorders.[21] Cognitive behavioural therapy requires a high level of training in the therapist, and has been adapted for children and adolescents suffering depression. A course of treatment is characterised by 8–12 weekly sessions in which the therapist and the child collaborate to solve current difficulties. The treatment is structured, and often directed by a manual. Treatment generally includes cognitive elements, such as the challenging of negativistic thoughts, and behavioural elements such as structuring time to engage in pleasurable activity.

Interpersonal therapy A standardised form of brief psychotherapy (usually 12–16 weekly sessions) primarily intended for outpatients with unipolar non-psychotic depressive disorders. It focuses on improving the patient's interpersonal functioning and identifying the problems associated with the onset of the depressive episode.[22] In children and adolescents, interpersonal therapy has been adapted for adolescents to address common adolescent developmental issues, for example separation from parents, exploration of authority in relationship to parents, development of dyadic interpersonal relationships, initial experience with the death of relative or friend, and peer pressure.

Substantive changes since last issue of Clinical Evidence

Tricyclic antidepressants Inclusion of one additional RCT into existing meta-analysis produced little change in estimate of effectiveness but narrowed the 95% confidence intervals.[7]

Selective serotonin reuptake inhibitors One new systematic review; no change in conclusion.[10]

Selective noradrenergic reuptake inhibitors One new systematic review; no change in conclusion.[10]

Tricyclic antidepressants Update on harms from treatment with tricyclic antidepressants from a systematic review in publication (P Hazell et al, personal communication, 2000).

Interpersonal therapy One additional RCT did not find a significant difference in recovery from interpersonal therapy compared with waiting list control.[16]

Long term outcome A 2 year follow up found no difference in long term outcomes between selected psychological treatments in adolescents with depression.[20]

REFERENCES

1. Costello EJ, Angold A, Burns BJ, et al. The Great Smoky Mountains Study of Youth. Goals, design, methods, and the prevalence of DSM-III-R disorders. *Arch Gen Psychiatry* 1996;53:1129–1136.
2. Costello EJ. Developments in child psychiatric epidemiology. *J Am Acad Child Adolesc Psychiatry* 1989;28:836–841.
3. Lewinsohn PM, Rohde P, Seely JR. Major depressive disorder in older adolescents: Prevalence, risk factors, and clinical implications. *Clin Psychol Rev* 1998;18:765–794.
4. Birmaher B, Ryan ND, Williamson DE, Brent DA. Childhood and adolescent depression: A review of the past 10 years, Part I. *J Am Acad Child Adolesc Psychiatry* 1996;35:1427–1439.
5. Geller B, Fox LW, Fletcher M. Effect of tricyclic antidepressants on switching to mania and on the onset of bipolarity in depressed 6- to 12-year-olds. *J Am Acad Child Adolesc Psychiatry* 1993; 32:43–50.
6. Hazell P, O'Connell D, Heathcote D, Henry D. Tricyclic drugs for depression in children and adolescents. In: The Cochrane Library 2000 Issue 1. Search date 1997; primary sources: Medline, Excerpta Medica, Cochrane trials database.
7. Bernstein, GA, Borchardt, CM, Perwien, AR, et al. Imipramine plus cognitive-behavioral therapy in the treatment of school refusal. *J Am Acad Child Adolesc Psychiatry* 2000;39:276–283.
8. Sallee FR, Vrindavanam NS, Deas-Nesmith D, Carson SW, Sethuraman G. Pulse intravenous clomipramine for depressed adolescents: Double-blind, controlled trial. *Am J Psychiatry* 1997;154: 668–673.
9. Avci A, Diler RS, Kibar M, Sezgin F. Comparison of moclobemide and placebo in young adolescents with major depressive disorder. *Ann Med Sci* 1999;8:31–40.
10. Williams JW, Mulrow CD, Chiquette E, Noel PH, Aguilar C, Cornell J. A systematic review of newer pharmacotherapies for depression in adults: Evidence report summary. *Ann Intern Med* 2000; 132:743–756. Search date 1998; primary sources Medline, Embase, Psyclit, Lilacs, Psyindex, Sigle, Cinahl, Biological Abstracts, Cochrane Controled Trials, hand searches, and personal contacts.
11. Geller B, Cooper TB, Zimerman B, et al. Lithium for prepubertal depressed children with family history predictors of future bipolarity: A double-blind, placebo-controlled study. *J Affect Disord* 1998;51:165–175.
12. Harrington R, Whittaker J, Shoebridge P, Campbell F. Systematic review of efficacy of cognitive behavioural therapies in childhood and adolescent depressive disorder. *BMJ* 1998;316:1559–1563. Search date 1997; primary sources Medline, Psychlit, Cochrane, and hand searches of reference lists, book chapters, conference proceedings, and relevant journals in the field.
13. Lewinsohn PM, Clarke GN. Psychosocial

treatments for adolescent depression. *Clin Psychol Rev* 1999;19:329–342.
14. Reinecke MA, Ryan NE, DuBois DL. Cognitive-behavioral therapy of depression and depressive symptoms during adolescence: A review and meta-analysis. *J Am Acad Child Adolesc Psychiatry* 1998;37:26–34.
15. Mufson L, Weissman MM, Moreau D, Garfinkel R. Efficacy of interpersonal psychotherapy for depressed adolescents. *Arch Gen Psychiatry* 1999;56:573–579.
16. Rossello J, Bernal G. The efficacy of cognitive-behavioral and interpersonal treatments for depression in Puerto Rican adolescents. *J Consult Clin Psychol* 1999;67:734–745.
17. Brent DA, Holder D, Kolko D, et al. A clinical psychotherapy trial for adolescent depression comparing cognitive, family, and supportive therapy. *Arch Gen Psychiatry* 1997;54:877–885.
18. Clarke GN, Rohde P, Lewinsohn PM, Hops H, Seeley JR. Cognitive-behavioral treatment of adolescent depression: Efficacy of acute group treatment and booster sessions. *J Am Acad Child Adolesc Psychiatry* 1999;38:272–279.
19. Fine S, Forth A, Gilbert M, Haley G. Group therapy for adolescent depressive disorder: a comparison of social skills and therapeutic support. *J Am Acad Child Adolesc Psychiatry* 1991;30:79–85.
20. Birmaher B, Brent DA, Kolko D, et al. Clinical outcome after short-term psychotherapy for adolescents with major depressive disorder. *Arch Gen Psychiatry* 2000;57:29–36.
21. Haaga DAF, Beck AT. Cognitive therapy. In: Paykel ES, ed. *Handbook of affective disorders.* Edinburgh: Churchill Livingstone, 1992;511–523.
22. Klerman GL, Weissman H. Interpersonal psychotherapy. In: Paykel ES, ed. *Handbook of affective disorders.* Edinburgh: Churchill Livingstone, 1992;501–510.

Philip Hazell
Conjoint Professor of Child and Adolescent Psychiatry/Director, Child and Youth Mental Health Service
University of Newcastle
New South Wales
Australia

Competing interests: PH has been paid a fee for speaking to general practitioners about the evidence for the treatment of depression in young people by Pfizer, the manufacturer of Sertraline.

Obsessive compulsive disorder

G Mustafa Soomro

QUESTIONS

INTERVENTIONS

Beneficial

Likely to be beneficial

To be covered in future issues of *Clinical Evidence*

Other forms of psychotherapy
Other drug monotherapies
Adjuvant/augmentation drug treatment
Psychosurgery
Electroconvulsive treatment
Treatment in children and adolescents

See glossary, p 57

Key Messages

- Three systematic reviews of RCTs have found that serotonin reuptake inhibitors improve symptoms. One double blind placebo substitution study found that most participants relapsed within weeks of stopping treatment.
- We found limited evidence from one RCT that sertraline is more effective than clomipramine at reducing symptoms. One systematic review and one RCT found no significant difference between clomipramine and other serotonin reuptake inhibitors. However, clomipramine has more adverse effects than selective serotonin reuptake inhibitors, particularly cholinergic and cardiac effects.
- One systematic review has found that behavioural therapy improves symptoms compared with relaxation. Two follow up studies found that improvement was maintained for up to 2 years.
- We found limited evidence from data pooling within a systematic review, and one RCT which found that cognitive therapy is as effective as behavioural therapy.
- One systematic review found no evidence of a difference between serotonin reuptake inhibitors and behavioural therapy.
- We found limited evidence from RCTs that behavioural therapy plus fluvoxamine is more effective than behavioural therapy alone.

Obsessive compulsive disorder

DEFINITION Obsessive compulsive disorder (OCD) is characterised by obsessions, compulsions, or both, that cause significant personal distress or social dysfunction, and that are not caused by drugs or physical disorder. **Obsessions** are defined as recurrent and persistent ideas, images, or impulses that cause pronounced anxiety and which the person perceives to be self produced. **Compulsions** are intentional repetitive behaviours or mental acts performed in response to obsessions or according to certain rules, and are aimed at reducing distress or preventing certain imagined dreaded events. Obsessions and compulsions are usually recognised as pointless and are resisted by the person. There are minor differences in the criteria for OCD between the third, revised third, and fourth editions of the *Diagnostic and Statistical Manual* (DSM-III, DSM-III-R, and DSM-IV).[1]

INCIDENCE/ PREVALENCE One national, community based survey of OCD in the UK (1993, n = 10 000) found prevalence to be 1% in men and 1.5% in women.[2] In the USA, the lifetime prevalence of OCD was found to be between 1.9–3.3% in 1984 (n = 18 500).[3] One international study found lifetime prevalence to be 3% in Canada, 3.1% in Puerto Rico, 0.3–0.9% in Taiwan, and 2.2% in New Zealand.[2]

AETIOLOGY/ RISK FACTORS Aetiology is unknown. Behavioural, cognitive, genetic, and neurobiological factors are implicated.[4–10]

PROGNOSIS One study that followed 144 people for an average of 47 years found that an episodic (see glossary, p 57) course was more common during the initial years (about 1–9 years), whereas a chronic (see glossary, p 57) course was more common afterwards.[11] Over time, the study found that 39–48% of people showed symptomatic improvement. A 1 year prospective cohort study found 46% of people to have an episodic course and 54% to have a chronic course.[12]

AIMS To improve symptoms and to reduce impact of illness on social functioning and quality of life.

OUTCOMES Severity of symptoms, adverse effects of treatment, and social functioning. The most commonly used instruments for measuring symptoms are the Yale–Brown obsessive compulsive scale and the National Institute of Mental Health's global obsessive compulsive scale, both of which are observer rated and well validated.[13–16] Most trials use a 25% decrease in Yale–Brown scale scores from baseline as indicative of clinically significant improvement. Some studies use a 35% reduction.[16]

METHODS *Clinical Evidence* update search and appraisal May 2000. We reviewed all identified systematic reviews and RCTs.

QUESTION What are the effects of treatments in adults?

OPTION SEROTONIN REUPTAKE INHIBITORS

Three systematic reviews and two subsequent RCTs have found good evidence that serotonin reuptake inhibitors (see glossary, p 57) are more effective than placebo in reducing symptoms. Apart from limited evidence from one RCT that sertraline is more effective than clomipramine, we

found no evidence of different efficacy for other serotonin reuptake inhibitors. One systematic review and two subsequent RCTs have found that serotonin reuptake inhibitors are more effective than other kinds of antidepressants. RCTs have found clomipramine to be associated with more adverse effects than selective serotonin reuptake inhibitors. One follow up study found that most people relapsed within a few weeks of stopping drug treatment.

Benefits: **Serotonin reuptake inhibitors versus placebo:** We found three systematic reviews and two subsequent RCTs. All found overall benefit of treatment compared with placebo.[17–21] The first review (search date 1994) identified nine RCTs of clomipramine (a non-selective serotonin reuptake inhibitor — see glossary, p 57) in 668 people, with mean treatment duration of 12 weeks. Two RCTs (n = 73) were in children, but the review did not give separate effect sizes.[18] This review found treatment to be more effective than placebo at reducing symptoms (WMD 1.31, 95% CI 1.15 to 1.47). The second review (search date not given) pooled data from eight placebo controlled RCTs of clomipramine (4 trials included in the first review; total of 1131 people with OCD).[18] It found clomipramine to be more effective than placebo (WMD 1.31, CI not given). The first review found fluoxetine, fluvoxamine and sertraline (selective serotonin reuptake inhibitors) to be more effective than placebo (fluoxetine: 1 RCT, 287 people; WMD 0.57, 95% CI 0.33 to 0.81; fluvoxamine: 3 RCTs, 395 people; WMD 0.57, 95% CI 0.37 to 0.77; sertraline: 3 RCTs, 270 people; WMD 0.52, 95% CI 0.27 to 0.77).[17] One subsequent double blind RCT compared fluoxetine 20 mg a day (n = 87) versus 40 mg a day (n = 89) versus 60 mg a day (n = 90) versus placebo (n = 84).[21] It found that people on all doses of fluoxetine improved significantly more than people on placebo (improvement on Yale–Brown scale, fluoxetine 20 mg 19.5%, 40 mg 22.1%, 60 mg 26.6%, placebo 3.3%, CI not given, all P *v* placebo $\leq$ 0.001). It also found a significant dose related response ($P < 0.001$). A second subsequent double blind RCT (164 people) found that sertraline was significantly more effective than placebo in reducing symptoms ($P < 0.01$, mean reduction on Yale–Brown scale 9 points with sertraline and 4 points with placebo, CI not given). The third review (search date 1997, 3 RCTs of 338 people) found paroxetine (a selective serotonin reuptake inhibitor) to be more effective than placebo over 12 weeks (WMD 0.48, 95% CI 0.24 to 0.72.[19,20] **Serotonin reuptake inhibitors versus each other:** The first review (85 people, three RCTs) found no significant difference in the improvement of obsessive compulsive symptoms between clomipramine and selective serotonin reuptake inhibitors (fluoxetine or fluvoxamine; WMD –0.04, 95% CI –0.43 to +0.35).[17] One subsequent double blind RCT of clomipramine (n = 82) versus sertraline (n = 86) found sertraline to be more effective (associated with a 8% greater mean reduction in obsessive compulsive symptoms; P = 0.036).[22] A second subsequent double blind RCT compared clomipramine (n = 65) with fluvoxamine (n = 68).[23] It found no significant difference in mean improvement in symptoms (improvement on Yale–Brown scale clomipramine 50.2% versus fluvoxamine 45.6%, CI and P not given). **Serotonin reuptake inhibitors versus other antidepressants:** The first systematic review identified seven RCTs comparing clomipramine with non-serotonin reuptake inhibitor antidepressants (147 people with OCD; 2 trials [n = 67] in children/adolescents without separate results).[17] This review found clomipramine to be more likely to reduce symptoms (WMD 0.65, 95% CI 0.36 to 0.92). One subsequent RCT of fluoxetine (n = 17) versus phenelzine (n = 19) versus placebo (n = 18) found the largest effect from fluoxetine (WMD not given, mean reduction in symptoms was 15% fluoxetine, 9% phenelzine, and 1% placebo).[24] A second subsequent double blind RCT compared sertraline (n = 79) with desipramine (n = 85) in people with concurrent OCD and major depressive disorder.[25] It found sertraline to be more effective at reducing obsessive compulsive and depressive symptoms. The response rate for improvement in obsessive compulsive symptoms (≥40% improvement on Y-BOCS) was 48% with sertraline compared with 31% with desipramine (CI not given, P = 0.01). There was no significant difference in response rate for depressive symptoms (≥50% improvement on Hamilton rating scale for depression) but the remission rate (defined as a score ≤7 on Hamilton rating scale for depression) was significantly better with sertraline (49% v 35%, CI not given, P = 0.04). **Serotonin reuptake inhibitors versus behavioural therapy:** We found weak evidence from the third systematic review, which included mixed method studies (number of studies and people not given).[19] This review found no significant difference between effect sizes of serotonin reuptake inhibitors and behavioural therapy (see glossary, p 57) when compared with placebo, but did not make direct comparisons.[19]

Harms: Sixteen RCTs in the second review found a greater incidence of adverse effects with serotonin reuptake inhibitors than placebo (RRI 54% for clomipramine, 11% for fluoxetine, 19% for fluvoxamine, and 27% for sertraline).[18] The third systematic review of controlled and uncontrolled studies found the withdrawal rate due to adverse effects to be 11% for clomipramine, 10% for fluoxetine, 13% for fluvoxamine, 9% for sertraline, and 11% for paroxetine.[19] Anticholinergic adverse effects (dry mouth, blurred vision, constipation, and urinary retention), cardiac adverse effects, drowsiness, dizziness, and convulsions (convulsions usually at doses > 250 mg/day) have been reported to be most common with clomipramine,[26–28] whereas selective serotonin reuptake inhibitors are associated with fewer adverse effects but more nausea, diarrhoea, anxiety, agitation, insomnia, and headache.[26,27] Both clomipramine and selective serotonin reuptake inhibitors were associated with weight change and sexual dysfunction.[26,28] The subsequent RCT comparing sertraline (n = 79) with desipramine (n = 85) found more people discontinued because of adverse effects with desipramine (26% *v* 10%, P = 0.009).[25] The subsequent RCT comparing clomipramine (n = 65) with fluvoxamine (n = 68) found a higher rate of discontinuation because of adverse effects associated with clomipramine (13.8% *v* 7.4%, significance not assessed).[23] One non-systematic review identified three prospective cohort studies and five surveys which found fluoxetine during pregnancy did not significantly increase the risk of spontaneous abortion of major malformation (figures not provided).[29] It included one prospective cohort study (n = 174) and three surveys which suggested similar outcomes from other selective serotonin reuptake inhibitors (sertraline, paroxetine, or fluvoxamine). One prospective cohort study (n = 55) found preschool age children exposed to fluoxetine *in utero* showed no significant differences from children not exposed in global IQ, language, or behaviour. It included no long term harms for the other selective serotonin reuptake inhibitors.

Comment: The first systematic review also identified two small RCTs, which found no difference in the effects of placebo and non-serotonin reuptake inhibitors (imipramine and nortriptyline).[17] One small, observer blinded RCT of fluvoxamine (n = 10) versus paroxetine (n = 9) versus citalopram (n = 11) found no significant differences in the effects of these drugs, but the study was too small to exclude a clinically significant effect.[30] **Duration and discontinuation of treatment:** Most RCTs assessed efficacy over 10–12 weeks.[28,31] One prospective, 1 year study found that further significant improvement occurred in the 40 week open label extension, with some continuing adverse effects.[32] One placebo substitution study of clomipramine found that 89% (16/18) of people relapsed within 7 weeks of placebo treatment.[33] **Effects on people without depression:** The first systematic review found that serotonin reuptake inhibitors reduced symptoms in people without depression (5 RCTs including 594 people; WMD 1.37, 95% CI 1.19 to 1.55).[17] **Factors predicting outcome:** Four RCTs found that people who did not respond to treatment had younger age of onset, longer duration of the condition, higher frequency of symptoms, co-existing personality disorders, and a greater likelihood of previous hospital admission. Predictors of good response were older age of onset, history of remissions, no previous drug treatment, more severe OCD, and either high or low score on the Hamilton Depression Rating Scale.[34–37] Two cohort studies of people with OCD found that poor response to serotonin reuptake inhibitors was predicted by concomitant schizotypal personality disorder (see glossary, p 57), by tic disorder (see glossary, p 57) and also by severe OCD with cleaning rituals (OR 4.9, 95% CI 1.1 to 21.2).[38,39] The non-systematic review of effects in pregnancy may have been systematic but did not make explicit how articles were selected.[29]

OPTION BEHAVIOURAL THERAPY AND COGNITIVE THERAPY

One systematic review found behavioural therapy is associated with greater symptom reduction than relaxation. The review found limited evidence of no significant difference in symptom reduction between cognitive therapy (see glossary, p 57) and behavioural therapy. We found limited evidence that behavioural therapy plus fluvoxamine is more effective than behavioural therapy alone. One RCT found no significant difference between cognitive therapy alone and cognitive therapy plus fluvoxamine. Two follow up studies found that after behavioural therapy, significant improvement was maintained for up to 2 years, but that some people required additional behavioural therapy.

Benefits: **Behavioural therapy versus relaxation:** We found one systematic review (search date not given), which pooled results from two RCTs (121 people with OCD, further characteristics not specified). It found evidence that behavioural therapy reduced symptoms more than relaxation (WMD 1.18, $P < 0.01$, CI not given; 88% of people in the relaxation group did worse than the average improvement on behavioural therapy).[18] **Behavioural therapy versus cognitive therapy:** The same systematic review pooled results from four RCTs (92 people with OCD, further characteristics not specified). It found no significant difference in reduction of symptoms between behavioural therapy and cognitive therapy (WMD –0.19, CI not available).[18] **Combination treatment:** We found weak evidence from one systematic review (search date 1997). It pooled data from mixed method studies (number of studies and people not given) and compared three different regimens with placebo: behavioural therapy plus serotonin reuptake inhibitors; behavioural therapy alone; and serotonin reuptake inhibitors alone. The review found similar reductions in symptoms, but did not make direct comparisons between treatments.[19] One RCT in 99 people in an outpatient setting compared behavioural therapy, cognitive therapy, behavioural therapy plus fluvoxamine, and cognitive therapy plus fluvoxamine.[40] It found no significant differences in outcomes on the Yale–Brown scale (mean reduction in symptoms 32% with behavioural therapy, 47% with cognitive therapy, 49% with behavioural therapy plus fluvoxamine, 43% with cognitive therapy plus fluvoxamine; 16 people per arm would allow detection of a 25% change in the Yale–Brown scale). One double blind RCT (49 people in a teaching hospital setting) found significantly greater improvement in symptoms with behavioural therapy plus fluvoxamine than with behavioural therapy plus pill placebo (88% *v* 60% achieved a ≥35% reduction on the Yale–Brown scale; RR 0.3, 95% CI 0.1 to 0.96; NNT 3).[41] **Maintenance of improvement:** One prospective follow up of 20 people with OCD (specific diagnostic criteria not given) from a 6 month RCT of behavioural therapy found that 79% maintained improvement in obsessive compulsive symptoms at 2 year follow up.[42] One prospective non-inception cohort study of behavioural therapy in 21 people with OCD (specific diagnostic criteria not given) found that after the initial 2 weeks of treatment, 68–79% maintained complete or much improvement in symptoms at 3 months' follow up.[43] In both studies, however, some people required additional behavioural therapy during the follow up period.

Harms: We found no evidence from RCTs or cohort studies of adverse effects from behavioural or cognitive therapy. Case reports have described unbearable and unacceptable anxiety in some people receiving behavioural therapy.

Comment: **Factors predicting outcome:** We found two RCTs of behavioural therapy (duration 2.5 months and 32 weeks; total 96 people) and two retrospective cohort studies (duration 1 year and 11 weeks; total 346 people).[44–47] These found poorer outcome to be predicted by initial severity, depression, longer duration, poorer motivation, and dissatisfaction with the therapeutic relationship. Good outcome was predicted by early adherence to 'exposure homework' (that is, tasks to be carried out outside regular therapy sessions involving contact with anxiety provoking situations), employment, living with one's family, no previous treatment, having fear of contamination, overt ritualistic behaviour, and absence of depression.[44–46] Good outcome for women was predicted by having a co-therapist (someone usually related to the person, who is enlisted to help with treatment outside regular therapy sessions; OR 19.5, 95% CI 2.7 to 139.3).[47] Two systematic reviews of drug, and behavioural, cognitive, and combination treatments for OCD are being prepared.

GLOSSARY

Behavioural therapy Consists of exposure to the anxiety provoking stimuli and prevention of ritual performance.
Chronic Continuous course without periods of remission since first onset.
Cognitive therapy Aims to correct distorted thoughts (such as exaggerated sense of harm and personal responsibility) by Socratic questioning, logical reasoning, and hypothesis testing.
Episodic Episodic course with periods of remission since first onset.
Non-selective serotonin reuptake inhibitor Clomipramine (also classed as a tricyclic antidepressant).
Schizotypal personality disorder Characterised by discomfort in close relationships, cognitive and perceptual distortions, and eccentric behaviour.
Selective serotonin reuptake inhibitors Fluoxetine, fluvoxamine, sertraline, paroxetine, citalopram.
Tic disorder Characterised by motor tics, vocal tics, or both.

Substantive changes since last issue of Clinical Evidence

Serotonin reuptake inhibitors One new RCT found significant improvement in obsessive compulsive symptoms with a range of doses of fluoxetine versus placebo.[21]
Serotonin reuptake inhibitors One new RCT found no significant difference in improvement in obsessive compulsive symptoms with fluvoxamine versus clomipramine. More people withdrew because of adverse events with clomipramine.[23]
Serotonin reuptake inhibitors One RCT found sertraline to be more effective at reducing obsessive compulsive symptoms compared with desipramine. More people withdrew because of adverse events with desipramine.[25]
Serotonin reuptake inhibitors One non-systematic review found limited evidence from cohort studies and surveys that fluoxetine in pregnancy does not increase risk for spontaneous abortion or major malformation. One cohort study and surveys suggest the same for other selective serotonin reuptake inhibitors. One long term cohort of fluoxetine found no evidence of an effect on IQ, language, or behaviour in preschool children exposed *in utero*.[29]

REFERENCES

1. American Psychiatric Association. *Diagnostic and statistical manual of mental disorders,* 4th ed. Washington, DC: American Psychiatric Association, 1994.
2. Bebbington PE. Epidemiology of obsessive–compulsive disorder. *Br J Psychiatry* 1998; 35(suppl):2–6.
3. Karno M, Golding JM, Sorenson SB, Burnam MA. The epidemiology of obsessive–compulsive disorder in five US communities. *Arch Gen Psychiatry* 1988;45:1094–1099.
4. Baer L, Minichiello WE. Behavior therapy for obsessive–compulsive disorder. In: Jenike MA, Baer L, Minichiello WE, eds. *Obsessive–compulsive disorders*. St Louis: Mosby, 1998.
5. Steketee GS, Frost RO, Rheaume J, Wilhelm S. Cognitive theory and treatment of obsessive–compulsive disorder. In: Jenike MA, Baer L, Minichiello WE, eds. *Obsessive–compulsive disorders*. St Louis: Mosby, 1998.
6. Alsobrook JP, Pauls DL. The genetics of obsessive–compulsive disorder. In: Jenike MA, Baer L, Minichiello WE, eds. *Obsessive–compulsive disorders*. St Louis: Mosby, 1998.
7. Rauch SL, Whalen PJ, Dougherty D, Jenike MA. Neurobiologic models of obsessive compulsive disorder. In: Jenike MA, Baer L, Minichiello WE, eds. *Obsessive–compulsive disorders*. St Louis: Mosby, 1998.
8. Delgado PL, Moreno FA. Different roles for serotonin in anti-obsessional drug action and the pathophysiology of obsessive–compulsive disorder. *Br J Psychiatry* 1998;35(suppl):21–25.
9. Saxena S, Brody AL, Schwartz JM, Baxter LR. Neuroimaging and frontal–subcortical circuitry in obsessive–compulsive disorder. *Br J Psychiatry* 1998;35(suppl):26–37.
10. Rauch SL, Baxter Jr. LR. Neuroimaging in obsessive–compulsive disorder and related disorders. In: Jenike MA, Baer L, Minichiello WE, eds. *Obsessive–compulsive disorders*. St Louis: Mosby, 1998.
11. Skoog G, Skoog I. A 40-year follow-up of patients with obsessive–compulsive disorder. *Arch Gen*

Psychiatry 1999;56:121–127.
12. Ravizza L, Maina G, Bogetto F. Episodic and chronic obsessive–compulsive disorder. *Depress Anxiety* 1997;6:154–158.
13. Goodman WK, Price LH, Rasmussen SA, et al. The Yale–Brown obsessive compulsive scale. I. Development, use, and reliability. *Arch Gen Psychiatry* 1989;46:1006–1011.
14. Insel TR, Murphy DL, Cohen RM, Alterman I, Kilts C, Linnoila M. Obsessive–compulsive disorder. A double-blind trial of clomipramine and clorgyline. *Arch Gen Psychiatry* 1983;40:605–612.
15. Goodman WK, Price LH, Rasmussen SA, et al. The Yale–Brown obsessive compulsive scale. II. Validity. *Arch Gen Psychiatry* 1989;46:1012–1016.
16. Goodman WK, Price LH. Rating scales for obsessive–compulsive disorder. In: Jenike MA, Baer L, Minichiello WE, eds. *Obsessive–compulsive disorders*. St Louis: Mosby, 1998.
17. Piccinelli M, Pini S, Bellantuono C, Wilkinson G. Efficacy of drug treatment in obsessive–compulsive disorder. A meta-analytic review. *Br J Psychiatry* 1995;166:424–443. Search dates 1975 to May 1994; primary sources Medline and Excerpta Medica-Psychiatry.
18. Abramowitz JS. Effectiveness of psychological and pharmacological treatments for obsessive–compulsive disorder: a quantitative review. *J Consult Clin Psychol* 1997;65:44–52. Search date not given; primary sources Medline and PsycLIT.
19. Kobak KA, Greist JH, Jefferson JW, Katzelnick DJ, Henk HJ. Behavioral versus pharmacological treatments of obsessive compulsive disorder: a meta-analysis. *Psychopharmacology (Berl)* 1998; 136:205–216. Search date May 1997; primary sources Medline, PsycINFO, Dissertations, and Abstracts International databases.
20. Kronig MH, Apter J, Asnis G, et al. Placebo controlled multicentre study of sertraline treatment for obsessive–compulsive disorder. *J Clin Psychopharmacol* 1999;19:172–176.
21. Tollefson GD, Rampey AH, Potvin JH, et al. A multicenter investigation of fixed-dose fluoxetine in the treatment of obsessive–compulsive disorder. *Arch Gen Psychiatry* 1994:51:559–567.
22. Bisserbe JC, Lane RM, Flament MF. A double blind comparison of sertraline and clomipramine in outpatients with obsessive–compulsive disorder. *Eur Psychiatry* 1997;12:82–93.
23. Mundo E, Maina G, Uslenghi C. Multicentre, double-blind, comparison of fluvoxamine and clomipramine in the treatment of obsessive–compulsive disorder. *Int Clin Psychopharmacol* 2000;15:69–76.
24. Jenike MA, Baer L, Minichiello WE, Rauch SL, Buttolph ML. Placebo-controlled trial of fluoxetine and phenelzine for obsessive–compulsive disorder. *Am J Psychiatry* 1997;154:1261–1264.
25. Hoehn-Saric R, Ninan P, Black DW, et al. Multcenter double-blind comparison of sertraline and desipramine for concurrent obsessive–compulsive and major depressive disorders. *Arch Gen Psychiatry* 2000;57:76–82.
26. British National Formulary. London: British Medical Association and Royal Pharmaceutical Society of Great Britain, 1999.
27. Trindade E, Menon D. Selective serotonin reuptake inhibitors differ from tricyclics antidepressants in adverse events (Abstract). Selective serotonin reuptake inhibitors for major depression. Part 1. Evaluation of clinical literature. Ottawa: Canadian Coordinating Office for Health Technology Assessment, August 1997 Report 3E. *Evid Based Ment Health* 1998;1:50.
28. Jenike MA. Drug treatment of obsessive–compulsive disorders. In: Jenike MA, Baer L, Minichiello WE, eds. *Obsessive–compulsive disorders*. St Louis: Mosby, 1998:469–532.
29. Goldstein DJ, Sundell K. A review of safety of selective serotonin reuptake inhibitors during pregnancy. *Hum Psychopharmacol Clin Exp* 1999; 14:319–324.
30. Mundo E, Bianchi L, Bellodi L. Efficacy of fluvoxamine, paroxetine, and citalopram in the treatment of obsessive–compulsive disorder: a single-blind study. *J Clin Psychopharmacol* 1997; 17:267–271.
31. Rauch SL, Jenike MA. Pharmacological treatment of obsessive compulsive disorder. In: Nathan PE, Gorman JM, eds. *Treatments that work*. New York: Oxford University Press, 1998:359–376.
32. Rasmussen S, Hackett E, DuBoff E, et al. A 2-year study of sertraline in the treatment of obsessive–compulsive disorder. *Int Clin Psychopharmacol* 1997;12:309–316.
33. Pato MT, Zohar-Kadouch R, Zohar J, Murphy DL. Return of symptoms after discontinuation of clomipramine in patients with obsessive–compulsive disorder. *Am J Psychiatry* 1988;145: 1521–1525.
34. Ravizza L, Barzega G, Bellino S, Bogetto F, Maina G. Predictors of drug treatment response in obsessive–compulsive disorder. *J Clin Psychiatry* 1995;56:368–373.
35. Cavedini P, Erzegovesi S, Ronchi P, Bellodi L. Predictive value of obsessive–compulsive personality disorder in antiobsessional pharmacological treatment. *Eur Neuropsychopharmacol* 1997;7:45–49.
36. Ackerman DL, Greenland S, Bystritsky A. Clinical characteristics of response to fluoxetine treatment of obsessive–compulsive disorder. *J Clin Psychopharmacol* 1998;18:185–192.
37. Ackerman DL, Greenland S, Bystritsky A, Morgenstern H, Katz RJ. Predictors of treatment response in obsessive–compulsive disorder: multivariate analyses from a multicenter trial of clomipramine. *J Clin Psychopharmacol* 1994;14: 247–254.
38. Mundo E, Erzegovesi S, Bellodi L. Follow up of obsessive–compulsive patients treated with proserotonergic agents (letter). *J Clin Psychopharmacol* 1995;15:288–289.
39. Alarcon RD, Libb JW, Spitler D. A predictive study of obsessive–compulsive disorder response to clomipramine. *J Clin Psychopharmacol* 1993;13: 210–213.
40. van Balkom AJ, de Haan E, van Oppen P, Spinhoven P, Hoogduin KA, van Dyck R. Cognitive and behavioral therapies alone versus in combination with fluvoxamine in the treatment of obsessive compulsive disorder. *J Nerv Ment Dis* 1998;186:492–499.
41. Hohagen F, Winkelmann G, Rasche-Ruchle H, et al. Combination of behaviour therapy with fluvoxamine in comparison with behaviour therapy and placebo. Results of a multicentre study. *Br J Psychiatry* 1998;35(suppl):71–78.
42. Marks IM, Hodgson R, Rachman S. Treatment of chronic obsessive–compulsive neurosis by in-vivo exposure. A two-year follow-up and issues in treatment. *Br J Psychiatry* 1975;127:349–364.
43. Foa EB, Goldstein A. Continuous exposure and complete response prevention in obsessive–compulsive neurosis. *Behav Ther* 1978;9:821–829.
44. Keijsers GP, Hoogduin CA, Schaap CP. Predictors of treatment outcome in the behavioural treatment of obsessive–compulsive disorder. *Br J Psychiatry* 1994;165:781–786.
45. De Araujo LA, Ito LM, Marks IM. Early compliance and other factors predicting outcome of exposure

for obsessive–compulsive disorder. *Br J Psychiatry* 1996;169:747–752.
46. Buchanan AW, Meng KS, Marks IM. What predicts improvement and compliance during the behavioral treatment of obsessive compulsive disorder? *Anxiety* 1996;2:22–27.
47. Castle DJ, Deale A, Marks IM, Cutts F, Chadhoury Y, Stewart A. Obsessive–compulsive disorder: prediction of outcome from behavioural psychotherapy. *Acta Psychiatr Scand* 1994;89:393–398.

G Mustafa Soomro
Honorary Research Fellow
Section of Community Psychiatry
St George's Hospital Medical School
London
UK

Competing interests: None declared.

Post-traumatic stress disorder

Jonathan Bisson

QUESTIONS

INTERVENTIONS

See glossary, p 64

Key Messages

Prevention

- One systematic review of RCTs found no evidence that debriefing prevents post-traumatic stress disorder (PTSD), and one RCT found that it was associated with an increased risk of PTSD at 1 year.
- We found conflicting evidence on the effects of multiple episode intervention. One small RCT found no evidence of benefit from multiple episode psychological intervention. Two small RCTs found that five sessions of either cognitive behavioural therapy or prolonged exposure are superior to supportive counselling for preventing PTSD in people with acute stress after a traumatic event.

Treatment

- Evidence from mainly small RCTs suggests benefit from psychological treatments compared with supportive counselling, relaxation therapy, or no treatment.
- One systematic review of mainly small RCTs has found that antidepressants reduce symptoms more than placebo. The only anxiolytic drug evaluated, alprazolam, was the least effective drug treatment. We found insufficient evidence on the effects of antipsychotic drugs or carbamazepine.

DEFINITION Post-traumatic stress disorder (PTSD) occurs after a major traumatic event. Symptoms include upsetting thoughts and nightmares about the traumatic event, avoidance behaviour, numbing of general responsiveness, increased irritability, and hypervigilance.[1]

INCIDENCE/ PREVALENCE One large cross sectional study in the USA found that one in 10 women and one in 20 men experience PTSD at some stage in their lives.[2]

AETIOLOGY/ RISK FACTORS Risk factors include major trauma such as rape, a history of psychiatric disorders, acute distress and depression after the trauma, lack of social support, and personality factors (such as neuroticism).[3]

PROGNOSIS One large cross sectional study in the USA found that over a third of sufferers continued to satisfy the criteria for a diagnosis of PTSD 6 years after diagnosis.[2] Cross sectional studies provide weak evidence about prognosis.

AIMS To reduce initial distress after a traumatic event; to prevent PTSD and other psychiatric disorders; to reduce levels of distress in the long term; and to improve function and quality of life.

OUTCOMES Presence or absence of PTSD and severity of symptoms. Scoring systems include impact of event scale and clinician administered PTSD scale.

METHODS *Clinical Evidence* update search and appraisal May 2000.

QUESTION What are the effects of preventive psychological interventions?

One systematic review of RCTs found no evidence that single episode interventions prevent PTSD, and one of these RCTs found an increased risk of PTSD at 1 year. We found conflicting evidence on the effects of multiple episode intervention from three RCTs. One found no significant evidence of benefit, the other two found that five episodes of cognitive behavioural therapy (see glossary, p 64) were superior to supportive counselling (see glossary, p 64).

Benefits: **Single episode intervention ("debriefing"):** We found one systematic review (search date 1997), which identified six RCTs comparing early single episode interventions ("debriefing") with no intervention in 462 people.[4] The trials used psychological debriefing or similar techniques (see glossary, p 64). The review found that more people treated with debriefing still had PTSD at 3–5 months but the difference was not significant (OR 1.5, 95% CI 0.7 to 3.1). One of the trials followed people for 1 year after debriefing and found that debriefing versus no treatment was associated with increased rates of PTSD (OR 2.9, 95% CI 1.1 to 7.5). **Multiple episode intervention:** We found no systematic review. We found three RCTs. The first RCT (151 people) compared 3–6 sessions of educational and cognitive behavioural techniques with no psychological intervention.[5] Intervention began at least 1 month after a road traffic accident. There were no significant differences in outcomes between groups. The second RCT (24 people) compared five sessions of cognitive behavioural therapy (see glossary, p 64) with five sessions of supportive counselling (see glossary, p 64) in people with acute stress disorder within 2 weeks of a road accident or industrial accident.[6] Cognitive behavioural therapy was associated with a large reduction in the number of people who met PTSD diagnostic criteria immediately after treatment (8% *v* 83% with supportive counselling, $P < 0.001$) and at 6 months (17% *v* 67% with supportive counselling, $P < 0.05$).[7] The third RCT (66 survivors of road accidents or non-sexual assault with acute stress disorder) evaluated five 90 minute sessions of prolonged exposure versus supportive counselling versus prolonged exposure plus anxiety management. Immediately after completion of treatment, significantly lower rates of PTSD were found in the prolonged exposure group (14%) and in the prolonged exposure plus anxiety management group (20%) compared with the supportive counselling group (56%). The differences were still significant at 6 month follow up (15% *v* 23% *v* 67%).[8]

Harms: Two trials of single episode intervention found an increased risk of subsequent psychological problems in people receiving the intervention however initial traumatic exposure had been higher in these people.[4]

Comment: The systematic review found that the overall quality of the studies was poor.[4] Problems included lack of blinding, failure to state loss to follow up, and lack of intention to treat analysis despite high withdrawal rates. We found one further RCT of cognitive behavioural therapy in French bus drivers who had been attacked.[9] The trial suggested that early intervention with cognitive behavioural therapy reduces anxiety levels at 6 month follow up. The trial will be fully evaluated for the next edition of *Clinical Evidence*.

QUESTION What are the effects of psychological treatments?

Mainly small RCTs found evidence of benefit from psychological treatments compared with supportive counselling, relaxation therapy (see glossary, p 64), or no treatment.

Benefits: We found one systematic review of psychological treatments for PTSD (search date not given, published in 1998, 17 RCTs, 690 people).[7] They compared a range of specific psychological treatments versus supportive treatment or no intervention. All trials found that psychological treatment was associated with a greater improvement in immediate outcome (using a composite score of PTSD symptoms, anxiety, and depression) compared with supportive counselling or no treatment (overall effect size immediately after treatment 0.54, 95% CI not stated). The difference was still evident at 1 year (overall effect size from 12 studies with long term follow up 0.53, CI not stated). **Cognitive behavioural treatments:** We found one systematic review (search date not given) and two subsequent RCTs.[7,10,11] The review identified 14 RCTs of cognitive behavioural treatments in people with PTSD. Although many were of poor quality, all described a positive effect compared with no treatment. One RCT ($n = 45$) identified in the review, evaluated three types of cognitive therapy and found that all were better than no treatment at 3 months (effect sizes compared with no treatment: stress inoculation 1.1, 95% CI 0.66 to 1.5; supportive counselling

0.55, 95% CI 0.17 to 0.94; prolonged exposure therapy 1.67, 95% CI 1.2 to 2.1).[12] One subsequent RCT (n = 87) compared exposure or cognitive therapy or both with relaxation therapy.[10] The trial found that all cognitive behavioural treatments reduced symptoms of PTSD more than relaxation therapy, immediately and at 3 months (at 3 months n = 53; no intention to treat analysis performed).[13] The second subsequent RCT (54 people) found that 39% continued to suffer from PTSD one year after 16 one hour sessions of imaginal exposure therapy or cognitive therapy. There was no difference in the prevalence of PTSD between the two treatment groups.[11] **Eye movement desensitisation and reprocessing (EMDR):** We found no systematic review. We found seven small RCTs (257 people in total) evaluating at least three sessions of EMDR (see glossary, p 64). Three found that EMDR was associated with reduced symptoms compared with no treatment.[10,14,15] One found that EMDR was associated with a greater reduction in symptoms compared with relaxation therapy and another found that EMDR reduced symptoms compared with active listening therapy.[15,16] One RCT (n = 36) found a non-significant treatment advantage with EMDR compared with a form of exposure therapy.[14] One RCT found evidence that EMDR was less effective than cognitive behavioural therapy.[17] Three trials compared standard EMDR with EMDR without eye movements.[18–20] Two found that both interventions were associated with a reduction in symptoms (no significant difference between reductions), and one found that standard EMDR was more effective.[18–20] **Affect management:** We found one RCT comparing psychotherapy plus drug treatment with or without affect management (see glossary, p 64) in 48 women. The trial found that symptom control was greater with affect management.[21] The dropout rate was high (31%) and the analysis was not by intention to treat. **Other psychological treatments:** We found one RCT (112 people), which found no significant difference between psychodynamic psychotherapy (see glossary, p 64), exposure therapy, and hypnotherapy (see glossary, p 64). However, all were slightly better than remaining on the waiting list (no treatment control). The trial did not quantify results.[22] **Inpatient treatment programme:** We found no RCTs. **Drama therapy:** See glossary, p 64. We found no RCTs.

Harms: The studies gave no information on harms. Overall, cognitive behavioural therapy seems well tolerated. However, there have been case reports in some individuals of imaginal flooding (a form of cognitive behavioural therapy) worsening symptoms, leading to calls for caution when assessing people for treatment.[23]

Comment: Most RCTs were of poor quality. We found no theoretical basis for the use of EMDR in people with PTSD.

QUESTION What are the effects of drug treatments?

One systematic review of mainly small RCTs has found that antidepressants versus placebo reduce symptoms more than placebo. One small RCT of alprazolam versus placebo found a small effect. We found insufficient evidence on the effects of antipsychotic drugs or carbamazepine.

Benefits: **Antidepressants and anxiolytics:** We found one systematic review of antidepressants and anxiolytics for PTSD and one subsequent RCT.[24] The review (search date July 1996) identified six placebo controlled trials in 242 people.[25] The effect size for PTSD from all trials and all drugs versus placebo was 0.41 (CI not available). Effect sizes for individual drugs (CI not available) were fluoxetine 0.77 (n = 64, 1 trial), phenelzine 0.39 (n = 63, two trials), tricyclic antidepressants 0.32 (n = 149, 3 trials), and alprazolam 0.25 (n = 16, 1 trial). The review also found that drug treatment reduced depression and anxiety. The subsequent RCT (187 people attending outpatients with PTSD from a variety of traumatic events) compared sertraline, a selective serotonin reuptake inhibitor, with placebo. Sertraline increased the response rate (53% with sertraline *v* 32% with placebo; P = 0.008), although the actual reduction in traumatic stress symptoms was not very large.[24] **Antipsychotic drugs:** We found no RCTs. **Carbamazepine:** We found no RCTs.

Harms: The trials gave no information on harms. Known adverse effects include the need for dietary restriction and possible hypertensive crisis with monoamine oxidase inhibitors, anticholinergic effects with tricyclic antidepressants, nausea and headache with SSRIs, and dependency with benzodiazepines.

Comment: Small trial sizes and different populations make it difficult to compare results. Other treatments or combinations of drug and psychological treatment await evaluation. It is difficult to interpret effect sizes in terms of clinical importance rather than statistical significance. Some categorise effect sizes of less than 0.5 as small; between 0.5 and 0.8 as medium; and greater than 0.8 as large.

GLOSSARY

Affect management Entails managing mood.

Cognitive behavioural therapy Covers a variety of techniques. *Imaginal exposure* entails exposure to a detailed account or image of what happened. *Real life exposure* involves confronting real life situations that have become associated with the trauma, and cause fear and distress. *Cognitive therapy* entails challenging distorted thoughts about the trauma, the self, and the world. *Stress inoculation* entails instruction in coping skills and some cognitive techniques such as restructuring.

Drama therapy Entails using drama as a form of expression and communication.

Eye movement desensitisation (EMDR) and reprocessing Entails asking the person to focus on the traumatic event, a negative cognition associated with it, and the associated emotions.[26] The person is then asked to follow the therapist's finger as it moves from side to side. We found no theoretical basis for this intervention.

Hypnotherapy Entails hypnosis to allow people to work through the traumatic event.

Jacobson's relaxation therapy A form of muscle relaxation that avoids any exposure to the traumatic event.

Psychodynamic psychotherapy Entails analysis of defence mechanisms, interpretations, and pre-trauma experiences.

Psychological debriefing A technique that entails detailed consideration of the traumatic event and the normalisation of psychological reactions.

Supportive counselling A non-directive intervention dealing with current issues rather than the trauma itself.

Substantive changes since last issue of Clinical Evidence

Preventive psychological interventions One new RCT found that five sessions of prolonged exposure or prolonged exposure with anxiety management resulted in lower rates of PTSD than supportive counselling;[8] conclusion unchanged.

Psychological treatments One new RCT found no difference in effect after 16 one hour sessions of imaginal exposure therapy or cognitive therapy; conclusion unchanged.[11]

Drug treatment One new RCT found sertraline more effective than placebo in reducing traumatic stress symptoms; conclusion unchanged.[24]

REFERENCES

1. American Psychiatric Association. *Diagnostic and statistical manual of mental disorders*. 4th ed. Washington: APA, 1994.
2. Kessler RC, Sonnega A, Bromet E, et al. Post-traumatic stress disorder in the national comorbidity survey. *Arch Gen Psychiatry* 1995;52:1048–1060.
3. O'Brien S. *Traumatic events and mental health*. Cambridge: Cambridge University Press, 1998.
4. Wessely S, Rose S, Bisson J. A systematic review of brief psychological interventions ('debriefing') for the treatment of immediate trauma related symptoms and the prevention of posttraumatic stress disorder. In: The Cochrane Library, issue 4, 1999. Oxford: Update Software. Search date 1996, primary sources Medline, Embase, Psychlit, Pilots, Biosis, Pascal, *Occup Health Saf*, CDSR and the Trials register of the Cochrane Depression, Anxiety and Neurosis Group; hand search of *J Trauma Stress*, and contact with experts.
5. Brom D, Kleber RJ, Hofman MC. Victims of traffic accidents: incidence and prevention of post-traumatic stress disorder. *J Clin Psychol* 1993;49: 131–140.
6. Bryant RA, Harvey AG, Basten C, Dang ST, Sackville T, Basten C. Treatment of acute stress disorder: a comparison of cognitive behavioural therapy and supportive counselling. *J Consult Clin Psychol* 1998;66:862–866.
7. Sherman JJ. Effects of psychotherapeutic treatments for PTSD: a meta-analysis of controlled clinical trials. *J Trauma Stress* 1998;11:413–436. Search date not given; primary sources Psychlit, ERIC, Medline, Cinahl, Dissertation Abstracts, Pilots Traumatic Stress Database.
8. Bryant RA, Sackville T, Dang ST, Moulds M, Guthrie R. Treating acute stress disorder: an evaluation of cognitive behavior therapy and supportive counselling techniques. *Am J Psychiatry* 1999;156:1780–1786.
9. Andre C, Lelord F, Legeron P, Reigner A, and Delattre A. Controlled study of outcomes after 6 months to early intervention of bus driver victims of aggression [in French]. *Encephale* 1997;23: 65–71.
10. Rothbaum BO. A controlled study of eye movement desensitization and reprocessing in the treatment of posttraumatic stress disordered sexual assault victims. *Bull Menninger Clin* 1997; 61:317–334.
11. Tarrier N, Sommerfield C, Pilgrim H, Humphreys L. Cognitive therapy or imaginal exposure in the treatment of post-traumatic stress disorder. *Br J Psychiatry* 1999;175:571–575.
12. Foa EB, Rothbaum BO, Riggs DS, et al. Treatment of posttraumatic stress disorder in rape victims: a comparison between cognitive-behavioural procedures and counselling. *J Consult Clin Psychol* 1992;59:715–723.
13. Marks I, Lovell K, Noshirvani H, et al. Treatment of posttraumatic stress disorder by exposure and/or cognitive restructuring: a controlled study. *Arch Gen Psychiatry* 1998;55:317–325.
14. Vaughan K, Armstrong MS, Gold R, et al. A trial of eye movement desensitization compared to image habituation training and applied muscle relaxation in post traumatic stress disorder. *J Behav Ther Exp Psychiatry* 1994;25:283–291.
15. Carlson JG, Chemtob CM, Rusnak K, Hedland NL, Muraoka MY. Eye movement desensitization and reprocessing (EMDR) treatment for combat-related posttraumatic stress disorder. *J Trauma Stress* 1998;11:3–24.
16. Scheck MM, Schaeffer JA, Gillette C. Brief psychological intervention with traumatized young women: The efficacy of eye movement desensitization and reprocessing. *J Trauma Stress* 1998;11:25–44.
17. Devilly GJ, Spence SH. The relative efficacy and treatment distress of EMDR and a cognitive-behavior treatment protocol in the amelioration of posttraumatic stress disorder. *J Anxiety Disord* 1999;13:131–157.
18. Renfrey G, Spates CR. Eye movement desensitization: a partial dismantling study. *J Behav Ther Exp Psychiatry* 1994;24:251–259.
19. Pitman RK, Orr SP, Altman B, Longpre RE, Poire RE, Macklin ML. Emotional processing during eye movement densensitisation and reprocessing therapy of Vietnam veterans with chronic posttraumatic stress disorder. *Compr Psychiatry* 1996;37:419–429.
20. Wilson SA, Becker LA, Tinker RH. Eye movement desensitization and reprocessing (EMDR) treatment for psychologically traumatized individuals. *J Consult Clin Psychol* 1995;63:928–937.
21. Zlotnick C, Shea T, Rosen K, et al. An affect-management group for women with posttraumatic stress disorder and histories of childhood sexual abuse. *J Trauma Stress* 1997;10:425–436.
22. Brom D, Kleber RJ, Defares PB. Brief psychotherapy of posttraumatic stress disorders. *J Consult Clin Psychol* 1989;57:607–612.
23. Pitman RK, Altman B, Greenwald E, et al. Psychiatric complications during flooding therapy for posttraumatic stress disorder. *J Clin Psychiatry* 1991;52:17–20.
24. Brady K, Pearlstein T, Asnis GM, et al. Efficacy and safety of sertraline treatment of posttraumatic stress disorder: a randomized controlled trial. *JAMA* 2000;283:1837–1844.
25. Penava SJ, Otto MW, Pollack MH, et al. Current status of pharmacotherapy for PTSD: an effect size analysis of controlled studies. *Depress Anxiety* 1997;4:240–242. Search date July 1994; primary sources Psychlit, Medline.
26. Shapiro, F. Eye movement desensitisation: a new treatment for post-traumatic stress disorder. *J Behav Ther Exp Psychiatry* 1989;20:211–217.

Jonathan Bisson

Consultant Liaison Psychiatrist, Cardiff and the Vale NHS Trust, Cardiff, UK

Competing interests: None declared.

Schizophrenia

Stephen M Lawrie and Andrew McIntosh

QUESTIONS

INTERVENTIONS

See glossary, p 82

Key Messages

- Most evidence is from systematic reviews of small brief RCTs that report different outcomes. There is a need for larger trials, over longer periods, with well designed end points including standardised, validated symptom scales.
- Systematic reviews of RCTs have found:
  - Chlorpromazine improves clinical outcomes, but adverse effects make it unacceptable to many people.
  - There is limited evidence of benefit from depot haloperidol decanoate compared with placebo.
  - The newer antipsychotic drugs olanzapine, quetiapine, risperidone, ziprasidone, and zotepine are as effective as standard antipsychotics and have different profiles of adverse effects.
  - Relapse rates are significantly reduced by continuing antipsychotic medication for at least 6 months after an acute episode and by family interven-

tions. Weaker evidence suggests that social skills training and cognitive behavioural therapy may also reduce relapse rates.
  - No intervention has been consistently found to reduce negative symptoms.

- RCTs have found:
  - Limited evidence that compliance therapy, family therapy, and behavioural therapy may improve adherence with antipsychotic medication.

DEFINITION Schizophrenia is characterised by the "positive symptoms" of auditory hallucinations, delusions, and thought disorder, and the "negative symptoms" of demotivation, self neglect, and reduced emotion.[1]

INCIDENCE/ PREVALENCE Onset of symptoms typically occurs in early adult life (average age 25 years) and is earlier in men than women. Prevalence worldwide is 2–4/1000. One in 100 people will develop schizophrenia in their lifetime.[2,3]

AETIOLOGY/ RISK FACTORS Risk factors include a family history (although no major genes have been identified); obstetric complications; developmental difficulties; central nervous system infections in childhood; cannabis use; and acute life events.[2] The precise contributions of these factors and ways in which they may interact are unclear.

PROGNOSIS About three quarters of people suffer recurrent relapse and continued disability, although outcomes were worse in the pretreatment era.[4] Outcome may be worse in people with insidious onset and delayed initial treatment, social isolation, or a strong family history; in people living in industrialised countries; in men; and in people who misuse drugs.[3] Drug treatment is generally successful in treating positive symptoms, but up to a third of people derive little benefit and negative symptoms are notoriously difficult to treat. About half of people with schizophrenia do not adhere to treatment in the short term. The figure is even higher in the longer term.[5]

AIMS To relieve symptoms and to improve quality of life, with minimal adverse effects of treatment.

OUTCOMES Severity of positive and negative symptoms; global clinical improvement; global clinical impression (a composite measure of symptoms and everyday functioning); rate of relapse; adherence to treatment; adverse effects of treatment.

METHODS *Clinical Evidence* update search and appraisal April 2000. We also searched The Cochrane Library, Issue 2, 2000. Most of the trials we found were small, short term, with many different outcome measures.[6] There were a large number of high quality recent systematic reviews. Therefore, if possible we focused primarily on systematic reviews at the expense of subsequent RCTs and included only the outcomes we thought were the most clinically relevant (because different treatments are associated with different benefits and harms, we used estimates of global effectiveness if they were available). We searched for placebo controlled studies for standard antipsychotic medication, and comparative studies for newer antipsychotics.

QUESTION What are the effects of drug treatments?

OPTION CHLORPROMAZINE

One systematic review of RCTs has found that chlorpromazine produces global improvement in the short and medium term.

Benefits: **Versus placebo:** We found one systematic review (updated 1999, 45 RCTs, 3116, mean dose of 511 mg/day, range 25–2000 mg/day).[7] Chlorpromazine was more effective than placebo in terms of psychiatrist rated global improvement by at least 50% (RR 1.3, 95% CI 1.1 to 1.4; NNT 7, 95% CI 5 to 10) and global severity (RR 1.5, 95% CI 1.1 to 2.0; NNT 5, 95% CI 4 to 8) in the short and medium term (up to 6 months).

Harms: The systematic review found that adverse effects include sedation (RR 2.4, 95% CI 1.7 to 3.3; NNH 6, 95% CI 4 to 8), acute dystonias (RR 3.1, 95% CI 1.3 to 7.6; NNH 24, 95% CI 14 to 77), parkinsonism (RR 2.6, 95% CI 1.2 to 5.4; NNH 10, 95% CI 8 to 16), weight gain (RR 4.4, 95% CI 2.1 to 9; NNH 3, 95% CI 2 to 5), skin photosensitivity (RR 5.2, 95% CI 3 to 10; NNH 7, 95% CI 6 to 10), dizziness caused by hypotension (RR 1.9, 95% CI 1.3 to 2.6; NNH 12, 95% CI 8 to 20), and dry mouth (RR 4, 95% CI 1.6 to 10; NNH 19, 95% CI 12 to 37).[7] Chlorpromazine was also associated with a non-significantly higher rate of seizures (RR 2.4, 95% CI 0.4 to 16) and blood dyscrasias (RR 2.0, 95% CI 0.7 to 6). We found no long term data on the risk of tardive dyskinesia or the rare but potentially fatal neuroleptic malignant syndrome. Despite the frequent adverse effects, people receiving active treatment were more likely to stay in trials than those receiving placebo in both the short and the medium term.

Comment: The review did not categorise symptoms as positive or negative as this information was rarely available from included trials. Relative risks and numbers needed to treat were based on 6 months' data.

OPTION DEPOT HALOPERIDOL DECANOATE

One systematic review has found limited evidence from one RCT that depot haloperidol decanoate is more effective than placebo.

Benefits: **Versus placebo:** We found one systematic review, updated in 1998, which identified two RCTs.[8] One RCT (22 people) comparing intramuscular depot haloperidol decanoate (mean dose 150 mg monthly) with placebo found that haloperidol decanoate was more likely to result in a "reduced need for medication" at four months (RR 2.6, 95% CI 1.1 to 5.6; NNT with 4 months' treatment 2, 95% CI 1 to 2).

Harms: Compared with placebo, fewer people receiving haloperidol left the trial early (RR 0.2, 95% CI 0.1 to 0.4; NNT 2, 95% CI 1 to 3).[8]

Comment: How "reduced need for medication" was measured was not described. Depot injection is believed to ensure adherence, but we found no evidence to support this belief.

OPTION DEPOT PIPOTHIAZINE PALMITATE

One systematic review has found limited evidence from two RCTs that there is no significant difference between depot pipothiazine palmitate and standard antipsychotic drugs.

Benefits: **Versus standard oral antipsychotic drugs:** We found one systematic review, updated in 1999, which identified two RCTs, both conducted in the 1970s, comparing intramuscular pipothiazine palmitate with normal treatment ("standard" oral antipsychotic drugs, chosen by physicians).[9] Neither found a significant difference between active treatment and control groups (first trial, 124 people: WMD in composite rating of psychotic symptoms at 18 months –3.1, 95% CI –7.3 to +1.2; second trial, 48 people: no quantified results available).

Harms: One trial (mean dose 90 mg per month) found that the number of people needing to take anticholinergic drugs for unspecified reasons was not significantly different for those taking the depot and for those on standard drugs (RR 0.9, 95% CI 0.7 to 1.1).[9] Meta-analysis combining the first and the second trial (mean dose 113 mg per month for 6 months) found no overall difference in the numbers of people leaving the trial early (25% in both groups, RR 1.0, 95% CI 0.5 to 1.9).

Comment: Several other depot preparations are commercially available in different countries, but we found even less evidence for their efficacy versus placebo or standard antipsychotic drugs.

OPTION LOXAPINE

One systematic review of 22 small, brief RCTs comparing loxapine and standard antipsychotic drugs found no significant difference in their benefits or harms.

Benefits: **Versus standard antipsychotic drugs:** We found one systematic review (updated in 1999, 22 RCTs, 1073 people), which compared loxapine (dose range 25 to 250 mg daily) with standard antipsychotic drugs, usually chlorpromazine.[10] It found no significant differences in global improvement (9 RCTs, 411 people; RR not improved 0.9, 95% CI 0.7 to 1.2).

Harms: The systematic review found no significant difference in adverse effects.[11]

Comment: All trials were conducted in the USA or India and none lasted longer than 12 weeks.

OPTION MOLINDONE

One systematic review of RCTs found no significant difference between molindone and standard antipsychotic drugs in benefits or harms, but the RCTs were short and of poor quality.

Benefits: **Versus standard antipsychotic drugs:** We found one systematic review of molindone versus standard antipsychotic drugs (updated 2000, 13 RCTs, 469 people).[10] It found no significant differences in global efficacy between molindone and standard antipsychotic drugs (4 RCTs, 150 people; RR no improvement 1.1, 95% CI 0.7 to 1.8).

Harms: No significant differences were found between molindone and standard antipsychotic drugs in terms of total numbers of adverse events. One trial found that the rate of confusion was higher in people taking molindone (RR 3.2, 95% CI 1.4 to 7.3). There were no significant differences in the rates of movement disorders between molindone and standard antipsychotic drugs. Weight loss was more frequent in those taking molindone (2 RCTs, 60 people; RR 2.8, 95% CI 1.1 to 7.0). Molindone was associated with less frequent weight gain than standard antipsychotic drugs (2 RCTs, 60 people; RR 0.4, 95% CI 0.1 to 1.0).

Comment: The RCTs in the review had methodological problems (in four trials it was unclear whether randomisation had been performed, 7/13 trials included people whose diagnosis was not operationally defined) and were brief (all lasted under 13 weeks). We found no reliable evidence comparing molindone with either placebo or new antipsychotic drugs.

OPTION PIMOZIDE

One systematic review of RCTs comparing pimozide with standard antipsychotic drugs found no significant difference in benefits or harms.

Benefits: **Versus standard antipsychotic drugs:** We found one systematic review (updated in 1999, 34 RCTs, 1278 people).[12] It identified trials including 1155 people comparing pimozide (mean dose 7.5 mg daily, range 1 to 75 mg daily) with a variety of standard antipsychotic drugs.[12] It found no significant differences in clinical global impression rates (3 RCTs, 206 people; RR 0.9, 95% CI 0.8 to 1.1).

Harms: Pimozide caused less sedation than standard antipsychotic drugs (RR 0.4, 95% CI 0.2 to 0.7; NNT 6, 95% CI 4 to 16), but was more likely to cause tremor (RR 1.6, 95% CI 1.1 to 2.3; NNH 6, 95% CI 3 to 44).

Comment: Sudden death has been reported in a number of people taking pimozide at doses over 20 mg daily, but we found no evidence that pimozide is more likely to cause sudden death than other antipsychotic drugs. The manufacturer recommends periodic ECG monitoring in all people taking more than 16 mg daily of pimozide and avoidance of other drugs known to prolong the QT interval on an electrocardiogram or cause electrolyte disturbances (other antipsychotics, antihistamines, antidepressants, and diuretics).

OPTION POLYUNSATURATED FATTY ACIDS

One systematic review found limited evidence from one small, brief RCT that polyunsaturated fatty acids compared with placebo reduced the subsequent use of antipsychotic medication.

Benefits: **Versus placebo:** We found one systematic review (updated 2000, 4 RCTs). It identified one relevant RCT (30 people) of fatty acid supplementation versus placebo.[13] The need at 12 weeks for subsequent antipsychotic medication was less in those receiving fish oil compared with those receiving placebo (RR 0.6, 95% CI 0.4 to 0.9). The review also found a slight difference in average symptom severity scores favouring fish oil (26 people; WMD −12.5, 95% CI −21.9 to −3.0).

Harms: The RCT did not find significant adverse events.

Comment: The single relevant RCT cited in the systematic review is an unpublished conference proceeding. Other RCTs considered only augmentation of antipsychotic treatment, which may be covered in a later issue of *Clinical Evidence.*

OPTION OLANZAPINE

Two systematic reviews of RCTs have found that olanzapine may be as effective as standard antipsychotic drugs and has fewer adverse effects. We found no evidence that olanzapine is more effective than other new antipsychotic drugs.

Benefits: We found three systematic reviews.[14–16] **Versus standard antipsychotic drugs:** The first review (updated 1999, 15 RCTs, 3282 people) compared olanzapine with standard antipsychotic drugs, usually haloperidol.[14] It found olanzapine 2.5–25 mg daily compared with standard antipsychotic drugs did not significantly reduce psychotic symptoms over 6–8 weeks (2778 people; RR of no important response defined as a 40% reduction on any scale: 0.9, 95% CI 0.76 to 1.06). The second review (search date 1998, 4 RCTs, 2914 people) found that olanzapine was associated with slightly greater treatment success than haloperidol on a composite measure of positive and negative symptoms.[15] We found one potentially relevant subsequent RCT comparing olanzapine with haloperidol.[17] It will be appraised for the next issue of *Clinical Evidence*. **Versus other new antipsychotic drugs:** The first review included one trial (84 people) comparing olanzapine with risperidone.[15] It found no evidence of a difference in effectiveness (RR no important clinical response by eight weeks 0.93, 95% CI 0.85 to 1.01). A third systematic review (180 people, 1 trial) comparing olanzapine with clozapine found no significant difference in effectiveness (RR no important clinical response 0.7, 95% CI 0.5 to 1.1).[16]

Harms: **Versus standard antipsychotic drugs:** Olanzapine compared with standard antipsychotic drugs did not significantly reduce the number of people who withdrew from the trials at 6–8 weeks (36% *v* 49%; RR 0.9, 95% CI 0.7 to 1.1) or at one year (83% *v* 90%; OR 0.9, 95% CI 0.86 to 1.02).[14] Olanzapine compared with standard antipsychotic drugs caused fewer extrapyramidal adverse effects (in heterogeneous data prone to bias), less nausea (2347 people; RR 0.7, 95% CI 0.6 to 0.9; NNT 25, 95% CI 14 to 85), vomiting (1996 people; RR 0.6, 95% CI 0.4 to 0.8; NNT 20, 95% CI 12 to 46), or drowsiness (2347 people; RR 0.8, 95% CI 0.7 to 0.9) than standard antipsychotic drugs.[14] Olanzapine was associated with a greater increase in appetite (1996 people; RR 1.7, 95% CI 1.4 to 2.0; NNH 10, 95% CI 7 to 15) and weight gain (heterogeneous data) than standard antipsychotic drugs.[14] **Versus other new antipsychotic drugs:** One RCT included in the first review (84 people) found that olanzapine compared with risperidone was associated with fewer extrapyramidal adverse effects (NNT 8), less parkinsonism (NNT 11) and less need for anticholinergic medication (NNT 8); but olanzapine caused more dry mouth (NNH 9) and greater weight gain (NNH 11).[14] RCTs (180 people) found olanzapine compared with clozapine was associated with less nausea (RR 0.1, 95% CI 0.01 to 0.8) and no significant change in the number of people complaining of movement disorders (RR 0.4, 95% CI 0.1 to 1.4).[16]

Comment: The results of the reviews are dominated by one large multicentre RCT reported by drug company employees. Benefits seem to be maximal at a dose of 15 mg daily, and higher doses may be associated with more harms. The results depended on the precise statistical test used. Those presented above are conservative estimates, which seem reasonable given the presence of heterogeneity and other possible biases. Some less conservative statistical methods indicate superior effectiveness for olanzapine compared with standard antipsychotic drugs.

OPTION QUETIAPINE

Two systematic reviews of RCTs and one subsequent RCT comparing quetiapine with standard antipsychotic drugs have found no significant differences in benefits, but significant reduction of some harms.

Benefits: **Versus standard antipsychotic drugs:** We found two systematic reviews, and one subsequent RCT.[15,18,19] The first review (search date 1998, 6 RCTs, 1414 people) identified two RCTs (809 people) comparing quetiapine with haloperidol and found no evidence of a difference in effectiveness on a composite measure of positive and negative symptoms.[15] The second (updated 1999, 7 RCTs, 2025 people), identified four trials comparing quetiapine (50–800 mg daily) with standard antipsychotic drugs, usually haloperidol.[18] No significant differences in global improvement were reported (310 people; RR no important improvement in mental state 1.1, 95% CI 0.8 to 1.5). The subsequent RCT (448 people) comparing quetiapine with haloperidol found no significant difference in improvement of global impression.[19]

Harms: The review found quetiapine caused less dystonia than standard antipsychotics (558 people; 1% *v* 5%; RR 0.2, 95% CI 0.1 to 0.9;

NNT 29, 95% CI 13 to 111) but no significant difference in the incidence of dry mouth (649 people; RR 2.5, 95% CI 0.7 to 9) or sleepiness (959 people; RR 1.4, 95% CI 0.8 to 2.5).[18,22] The subsequent RCT found no significant difference in overall adverse effects.[18] It did find significantly less extrapyramidal effects with quetiapine (62% v 14%).[19]

Comment: The evidence comes from a small number of short term trials that had substantial withdrawal rates and did not conduct intention to treat analyses. The Cochrane review has been substantially amended subsequent to our search date; the amendments will be included in the next issue of *Clinical Evidence*.[20]

OPTION RISPERIDONE

Two systematic reviews of RCTs comparing risperidone with standard antipsychotic drugs (mainly haloperidol) have found limited evidence that risperidone may be more effective than standard antipsychotic drugs and good evidence that at lower doses it has fewer adverse effects.

Benefits: **Versus standard antipsychotic drugs:** We found two systematic reviews, and one additional RCT.[15,21,22] Both systematic reviews found that risperidone was more effective than haloperidol. The first review (updated 1997, 14 RCTs, 3401 people) found that, at 12 weeks, risperidone (mean daily dose range 6.1–12 mg) was more effective than standard antipsychotic drugs, usually haloperidol.[21] Outcome was "clinical improvement," variably defined but usually a 20% reduction in general symptoms (2171 people; 11 RCTs, RR no improvement 0.8, 95% CI 0.7 to 0.9; NNT 10, 95% CI 7 to 16). No benefit was observed for the outcome of global clinical impression. The second review (search date 1998, 9 RCTs, 2215 people) found that risperidone was associated with slightly greater success than haloperidol on a composite measure of positive and negative symptoms.[15] The additional RCT (99 people) comparing a range of doses of risperidone with haloperidol found no overall significant difference in global outcome.[22] **Versus other new antipsychotic drugs:** See olanzapine, p 82. One systematic review found no significant difference between risperidone and clozapine for outcomes such as "improvement in mental state" but only 135 people were involved in the three RCTs.

Harms: The systematic review found that risperidone compared with standard antipsychotic drugs caused no significant change in the number of people who withdrew from treatment (2166 people; RR 0.8, 95% CI 0.6 to 1.1). People taking risperidone developed fewer extrapyramidal effects (2279 people; RR 0.6, 95% CI 0.5 to 0.7; NNT 5, 95% CI 5 to 10), required less antiparkinsonian medication (2436 people; RR 0.6, 95% CI 0.5 to 0.7; NNT 7, 95% CI 5 to 10), and were less likely to develop daytime somnolence (2098 people; RR 0.9, 95% CI 0.7 to 0.99; NNT 22, 95% CI 11 to 500). Risperidone was associated with greater weight gain (1652 people; RR 1.4, 95% CI 1.1 to 1.7; NNH 13, 95% CI 8 to 36).[21] The additional RCT found no overall significant difference in the rate of adverse effects between risperidone and haloperidol.[22]

Comment: The reported benefits in the first review over standard antipsychotic drugs were marginal and it found evidence of publication bias.[21]

Sensitivity analyses found that benefits in clinical improvement and continuing treatment of risperidone compared with standard antipsychotic drugs were no longer significant if studies using more than 10 mg haloperidol daily were excluded.[21] This loss of significance could be because of loss of power when studies were excluded. Exclusion of the higher dosage studies did not remove the difference in rate of extrapyramidal adverse effects.[21]

OPTION ZIPRASIDONE

One systematic review of RCTs comparing ziprasidone with standard antipsychotic drugs found no significant difference in mental state improvement but did find a different profile of adverse effects.

Benefits: We found one systematic review (updated 1999, 7 RCTs, 824 people) **Versus standard antipsychotics:** It identified four RCTs of ziprasidone versus standard antipsychotic drugs.[23] It found no significant differences in mental state improvement in different trials (301 people; RR no important improvement in mental state 0.9, 95% CI 0.7 to 1.0).

Harms: **Versus standard antipsychotics:** The review found no clear difference in total adverse events between ziprasidone and haloperidol.[23] Ziprasidone was less likely to cause akathisia in the short term (438 people; RR 0.3, 95% CI 0.2 to 0.6; NNT 8, 95% CI 5 to 18) or in the long term (301 people; RR 0.3, 95% CI 0.1 to 0.7, NNT 9, 95% CI 5 to 21), and less likely to cause acute dystonia (438 people; RR 0.4, 95% CI 0.2 to 0.9, NNT 16, 95% CI 9 to 166). Ziprasidone was more likely to produce nausea and vomiting in both the short (306 people; RR 3.6, 95% CI 1.8 to 7; NNT 5, 95% CI 4 to 8) and in the long term (301 people; RR 2.1, 95% CI 1 to 4, NNT 9, 95% CI 5 to 33). Intramuscular ziprasidone was significantly more likely to be associated with injection site pain than haloperidol (306 people; RR 5.3, 95% CI 1.3 to 22; NNT 12, 95% CI 7 to 27).

Comment: The duration of RCTs was less than 6 weeks. Most reported a withdrawal rate of over 20% and no RCT clearly described adequate precautions for the blinding of treatment allocation. We found no evidence comparing ziprasidone with other new antipsychotic drugs.

OPTION ZOTEPINE

One systematic review of small, brief RCTs that compared zotepine with standard antipsychotic drugs found weak evidence that zotepine reduced a standard symptom severity score and had fewer adverse effects. This finding was not robust as removal of a single RCT alters the conclusion. We found no evidence comparing zotepine with other new antipsychotic drugs.

Benefits: **Versus standard antipsychotic drugs:** We found one systematic review (updated 1999, 10 RCTs, 537 people). The systematic review included eight RCTs comparing zotepine (75–450 mg daily) with a variety of standard antipsychotic drugs.[24] Zotepine was more likely than standard antipsychotic drugs to bring about "clinically important improvement" as defined by a pre-stated cut off point on the Brief Psychiatric Rating Scale (356 people; 4 RCTs, RR 1.25, 95% CI 1.1 to 1.4; NNT 7, 95% CI 4 to 22).

Harms: The review found zotepine caused less akathisia (396 people; RR 0.7, 95% CI 0.6 to 0.9; NNT 8, 95% CI 5 to 34), dystonia (70 people; RR 0.5, 95% CI 0.2 to 0.9; NNT 4, 95% CI 2 to 56), and rigidity (164 people; RR 0.6, 95% CI 0.4 to 0.9; NNT 7, 95% CI 4 to 360) than standard antipsychotic drugs.[24]

Comment: All but one trial were of 12 weeks or less duration and all were conducted in Europe. Only one RCT favoured zotepine over standard antipsychotic drugs and removal of this RCT from the analysis changed the result from a significant to a non-significant effect. Two RCTs found abnormal ECG results in people taking zotepine, but few additional details were given. We found too few trials to compare zotepine reliably with other new antipsychotics.

OPTION CLOZAPINE

One systematic review of RCTs has found that clozapine is more effective than standard antipsychotic drugs. It is, however, associated with potentially fatal blood dyscrasias. A second systematic review of RCTs found no strong evidence about the effectiveness or safety of clozapine compared with new antipsychotic drugs.

Benefits: **Versus standard antipsychotics:** We found one systematic review (updated in 1998, 31 RCTs, 2530 people; 73% men).[25] Compared with standard antipsychotics such as chlorpromazine and haloperidol, clozapine was associated with greater clinical improvement both in the short term (4–10 weeks, 14 RCTs, 1131 people; RR no important improvement 0.7, 95% CI 0.7 to 0.8; NNT 6, 95% CI 5 to 7) and the long term (heterogeneous data). **Versus new antipsychotics:** We found one systematic review (updated 2000, 8 RCTs) that compared clozapine with the new antipsychotics, including olanzapine and risperidone.[26] It found no significant difference in efficacy, but the number of people studied was too small to rule out a clinically important difference.

Harms: **Versus standard antipsychotics:** Clozapine was more likely to cause hypersalivation (1419 people; RR 3.0, 95% CI 1.8 to 4.7; NNH 3), temperature increases (1147 people; RR 1.8, 95% CI 1.2 to 2.7; NNH 11), and sedation (1527 people; RR 1.2, 95% CI 1.1 to 1.4; NNH 10), but less likely to cause dry mouth (799 people; RR 0.4, 95% CI 0.3 to 0.6; NNT 6) and extrapyramidal adverse effects (1235 people; RR 0.7, 95% CI 0.5 to 0.9; NNT 6).[26] The review found blood problems occurred more frequently with clozapine than with standard antipsychotics (1293 people; AR 3.6% *v* 1.9%; ARI 1.7, 95% CI 0.9 to 3.2).[25] In a large observational case series leucopenia was reported in 3% of 99 502 people over 5 years. However, it found monitoring white cell (neutrophil) counts was associated with a lower than expected rate of cases of agranulocytosis (382 *v* 995, AR 0.38% *v* 1%) and deaths (12 *v* 149).[27] Dyscrasias were more common in younger people in a single RCT included in the first systematic review (21 people; RR 5.4, 95% CI 10 to 162; NNH 2.5).[25,28] Despite the requirement for regular blood tests, fewer people withdrew from treatment with clozapine in the long term (1513 people; RR 0.8, 95% CI 0.6 to 0.9; NNH 3).[25] **Versus new antipsychotics:** Compared with new antipsychotic drugs (mainly risperidone), clozapine was less likely to cause extrapyramidal adverse effects (305 people; RR 0.3, 95% CI 0.1 to 0.6; NNT 6, 95% CI 4 to 9). Clozapine may also be less likely to cause dry mouth and more likely to cause fatigue, nausea, dizziness, hypersalivation and hypersomnia, but these findings were from one or at most two trials.[26] The second review found no difference in rates of blood dyscrasias between clozapine and the new antipsychoytics, but the number of people studied was too small (558) to rule out a clinically important difference.[26] It found that compared with new antipsychotics, people on clozapine tended to be more satisfied with their treatment, but also to withdraw from trials more easily.[26]

Comment: Some of the benefits of clozapine were more apparent in the long term, depending on which drug was used for comparison in the trials.

QUESTION **Which interventions reduce relapse rates?**

OPTION **CONTINUED TREATMENT WITH ANTIPSYCHOTIC DRUGS**

One systematic review of follow up studies has found that continuing antipsychotic medication for at least 6 months after an acute episode significantly reduces relapse rates, and that some benefit of continuing treatment is apparent for up to 2 years. We found no evidence of a difference in relapse rates between standard antipsychotic drugs, but a systematic review of RCTs has found that relapse rates are lower with clozapine.

Benefits: **Versus no treatment or placebo:** We found two systematic reviews.[6,29] Both found evidence that continued treatment was beneficial for prevention of relapse. One review (search date not given, 66 studies, 4365 people taking antipsychotic drugs, mean dose 630 mg chlorpromazine equivalents a day, mean follow up of 6.3 months) included 29 controlled trials with a mean follow up of 9.7 months.[29] It found significantly lower relapse in 1224 people maintained on treatment compared with 1224 withdrawn from treatment (16.2% *v* 51.5%; ARR 35%, 95% CI 33% to 38%; NNT 3, 95% CI 2.6 to 3.1). Over time, the relapse rate in people maintained on antipsychotic treatment approached that in those withdrawn from treatment, but was still lower in those on treatment at 2 years (ARR 22%; NNT 5). The other review (updated in 1997) found that relapse rates over 6–24 months were significantly lower on chlorpromazine than placebo (3 heterogeneous RCTs; RR 0.7, 95% CI 0.5 to 0.9; NNT 3, 95% CI 2.5 to 4).[6] **Choice of drug:** We found eight systematic reviews which found that the choice of drug or preparation did not seem to affect relapse rates. The first (search date 1995) identified six RCTs comparing oral with depot fluphenazine (see table 1, p 85).[30] A second (updated in 1998) identified seven RCTs comparing haloperidol decanoate with other depot antipsychotics.[8] A third (updated in 1999) identified eight RCTs comparing flupenthixol decanoate with other depot antipsychotics.[31] A fourth (updated in 1999) identified seven RCTs comparing pipothiazine palmitate with other depots and two RCTs comparing pipothiazine palmitate with oral antipsychotics.[9] A fifth (updated in 1999) identified one RCT comparing fluspirilene decanoate with oral chlorpromazine and three studies comparing fluspirilene decanoate with other depot preparations.[32] A sixth (updated in 1999) found one RCT comparing perphenazine enanthate with clopenthixol decanoate.[33] The reviews comparing pimozide and olanzapine versus typical antipsychotic drugs also found no significant difference in relapse rates.[12–14] The number of people studied was too small to rule out clinically important differences. One systematic review comparing clozapine with standard antipsychotic drugs (search date 1998) found that relapse rates up to 12 weeks were significantly lower with clozapine (19 RCTs; RR 0.6, 95% CI 0.5 to 0.8; NNT 20).[25] Another systematic review found that significantly fewer people taking depot zuclopenthixol decanoate relapsed over 12 weeks to 1 year compared with people taking other depot preparations (3 RCTs, 296 people; RR 0.7, 95% CI 0.6 to 1.0; NNT 9, 95% CI 5 to 53).[34]

Harms: Mild transient nausea, malaise, sweating, vomiting, insomnia, and dyskinesia were reported in an unspecified number of people after sudden drug cessation, but were usually acceptable with gradual dose reduction.[35] Annual incidence of tardive dyskinesia was 5%.[34]

Comment: In the systematic review of continued versus withdrawal of treatment, meta-analysis of the 29 controlled trials gave similar results to those obtained when all 66 studies were included (ARR 37%, NNT 3).[34] The review was weakened because all RCT results were used rather than weighted comparisons, no length of time was given since the last acute episode, and no distinction was made between people experiencing a first episode and those with chronic illness.[34] Some clinicians use depot antipsychotic medication in selected people to ensure adherence with medication. We found no evidence from RCTs to support this practice.

OPTION FAMILY INTERVENTIONS

One systematic review of RCTs has found that family intervention significantly reduces relapse rates compared with usual care.

Benefits: We found one systematic review (updated 1999, 13 RCTs) and one additional RCT comparing family interventions with usual care.[36,37] Family interventions consisted mainly of education about the illness and training in problem solving over at least six weekly sessions. Three of the trials included substantial proportions of people experiencing their first episode. Family interventions significantly reduced relapse rates at 12 and 24 months. At 12 months, the risk of relapse was reduced (6 RCTs, 516 people; RR 0.7, 95% CI 0.5 to 1.0), such that seven families would have to be treated to avoid one additional relapse (and likely hospitalisation) in the family member with schizophrenia (NNT 7, 95% CI 4 to 14).[38] We found one potentially relevant additional RCT of family interventions compared with psychoeducation.[39] It will be assessed for the next issue of *Clinical Evidence*.

Harms: No harms were reported, although illness education could possibly have adverse consequences on morale and outlook.[38]

Comment: These results are likely to overestimate treatment effect because of the difficulty of blinding people and investigators and the likelihood of publication bias.[36] The trend over time is for results to tend to the null. The mechanism for the effects of family intervention remains unclear. It is thought to work by reducing "expressed emotion" (hostility and criticism) in relatives of people with schizophrenia, but may act through improved adherence to medication. The time consuming nature of this intervention, which must normally take place at evenings or weekends, can limit its availability. It cannot be applied to people who have little contact with home based carers.

OPTION SOCIAL SKILLS TRAINING

Limited evidence from RCTs suggests that social skills training may reduce relapse rates.

Benefits: We found one non-systematic review and meta-analysis of 27 RCTs (search date not given) comparing social skills training with usual care.[40] The trials were mainly in men admitted to hospital, not all of whom had schizophrenia, using different techniques that generally included instruction in social interaction. Four studies provided quantitative information, of which three defined relapse as rehospitalisation. Social skills training significantly reduced relapse rates (WMD 0.47). However, sensitivity analysis indicated that five null results (in studies not identified by a search) would render the difference non-significant. One systematic review (search date 1988) identified 73 RCTs in people with a variety of psychiatric disorders and found similar results, but suggested that motivation was an important predictor of benefit from treatment.[41]

Harms: None reported.

Comment: Many of the trials simultaneously compared the effects of other interventions (medication, education), so the effects of individual interventions are difficult to assess. Overall, it remains uncertain whether people at different stages of illness and function require different approaches. Selected people may benefit even from interventions of short duration.

OPTION COGNITIVE BEHAVIOURAL THERAPY

Limited evidence from RCTs suggests that cognitive behavioural therapy may reduce relapse rates.

Benefits: We found one systematic review (search date 1998, 4 small RCTs) comparing cognitive behavioural therapy plus standard care with standard care alone.[42] All trials incorporated the challenging of key beliefs, problem solving, and enhancement of coping. Relapse rates were significantly reduced in the short, medium, and long term. In the long term (up to 18 months), cognitive behavioural therapy plus standard care reduced the risk of relapse (3 RCTs, 183 people; RR 0.7, 95% CI 0.5 to 0.9; NNT 6, 95% CI 3 to 30).

Harms: None reported.

Comment: None of the three trials contributing long term results were blinded, and each concentrated on different clinical issues — symptoms, adherence to treatment, or general rehabilitation. The fourth trial blinded outcome raters and included an additional supportive psychotherapy control group. It found non-significantly lower relapse rates with cognitive behavioural therapy (1 RCT, 59 people; RR 0.6, 95% CI 0.2 to 2.1).

QUESTION **Which interventions are effective in people resistant to standard treatment?**

One systematic review of RCTs has found clozapine to benefit people who are resistant to standard treatment.

Benefits: **Clozapine:** We found one systematic review (updated 1998, 6 RCTs) comparing clozapine with standard antipsychotic drugs in people who were resistant to standard treatment.[25] Clozapine achieved improvement both in the short term (6–12 weeks: 370 people; 4 RCTs, RR for no improvement compared with standard antipsychotic drugs 0.7, 95% CI 0.6 to 0.8; NNT 5) and in the longer term (12–24 months: 648, 2 RCTs, RR 0.8, 95% CI 0.6 to 1.0). There was no difference in relapse rates in the short term. **Other interventions:** We found no good evidence on the effects of other interventions in people resistant to standard treatment.

Harms: See harms of clozapine, p 75.

Comment: Trials are under way to clarify the mode of action of cognitive behavioural therapy and establish its effects in people who are resistant to standard treatments.

QUESTION **Which interventions improve adherance to antipsychotic medication?**

OPTION **COMPLIANCE THERAPY**

We found limited evidence from three RCTs that compliance therapy (see glossary, p 82) may increase adherence with antipsychotic medication.

Benefits: We found no systematic review. We found one RCT of compliance therapy versus supportive counselling, that included 47 people with acute psychoses, although the majority fulfilled criteria for schizophrenia or had been admitted with the first episode of a psychotic illness.[38,43] People treated with compliance therapy were significantly more likely to attain at least passive acceptance of antipsychotic medication compared with people who received non-specific counselling, both immediately after the intervention (OR 6.3, 95% CI 1.6 to 24.6) and at six months follow up (OR 5.2, 95% CI 1.5 to 18.3). At 18 months (for an extended sample of 74 people) a significant improvement on a seven point scale of medication adherence was found for people treated with compliance therapy (mean difference 1.4, 95% CI 0.9 to 1.6).

Harms: None reported.

Comment: Other studies have examined the potential benefits of compliance therapy but either did not employ a standardised measure of adherence or adherence was not rated in a blind fashion. The RCT above requires independent replication. About one third of each group did not complete the trials and missing data are estimated from the mean scores in each group. Calculation of NNTs was not possible due to missing data.

OPTION FAMILY THERAPY

Limited evidence from three RCTs suggests that family therapy is an effective intervention for improving adherence with antipsychotic medication.

Benefits: We found no systematic review. We found three RCTs of family therapy in schizophrenia that directly assessed its impact on adherence to antipsychotic medication.[39,44,45] The first trial, conducted in the UK, compared family therapy with individual supportive therapy in 32 people recently discharged from hospital who all had at least one parent who exhibited high "expressed emotion".[39] People were followed up for six months. Those receiving family therapy were significantly more likely to take at least half of their prescribed antipsychotic dose than those receiving supportive therapy (ARI 0.54, NNT 2, 95% CI 2 to 5) as judged by tablet counts, reports from people with schizophrenia, their family, and blood levels. The second and third RCTs were conducted in China and used comparison with standard care only. The two trials may have included some or all of the same people. The first of these (63 people) measured adherence as "compliance with medication for at least 75% of the non-hospitalised follow up period".[44] The trial found no advantage of family therapy over standard care using the numbers of people in each group compliant with 50% of their medication dose, or when using the months of medication as an outcome measure. The third RCT was in 78 men with schizophrenia admitted to hospital for the first time.[45] Adherence was measured according to a criterion of "people taking at least 33% of the dose prescribed at the time of the index discharge for at least six days per week". The trial found an increase in medicated adherence with family therapy compared with standard care (ARI 0.23; NNT 5, 95% CI 3 to 34).

Harms: None reported.

Comment: The first trial was conducted in the UK and found that family therapy also improved attendance at clinic appointments. Both of the Chinese studies refer to the unique family structure in China. How adherence to medication was judged is unclear, but appears to have been rated blind to treatment allocation.

OPTION PSYCHOEDUCATIONAL THERAPY

Two RCTs have found that psychoeducational therapy has no significant effect on adherence to antipsychotic medication.

Benefits: We found no systematic review. **Versus usual treatment:** We found one RCT (36 men) comparing psychoeducation versus behavioural therapy versus usual treatment.[46] It found no significant difference between psychoeducation and usual treatment (quantified results not presented). **Versus behavioural therapy**: We found three RCTs.[46–48] One RCT compared behavioural therapy with psychoeducation (36 men) and with usual treatment.[46] The behavioural training method comprised being told the importance of complying with antipsychotic medication and instructions on how to take medication. Each participant was given a self-monitoring spiral calendar, which featured a dated slip of paper for each dose of antipsychotic. Adherence was estimated by pill counts. After three months fewer people had high pill adherence after psychoeducation compared with behaviour therapy (3/11 *v* 8/11 had pill adherence scores of 80% measured by pill counts). The second RCT (39 people) compared a behavioural intervention given individually, a behavioural intervention involving the person with schizophrenia and their family, and a psychoeducational intervention.[47] The behavioural intervention consisted of specific written guidelines, and oral instructions, given to people to use a pill box consisting of 28 compartments for every medication occasion during a week. The behavioural intervention, when given to the individual and their family, also consisted of instructions for the family member to compliment the person with schizophrenia for taking their prescribed medication. The primary outcome measure was pill count at two months. Medication adherence was more likely with behavioural interventions than with psychoeducation (over 90% adherence at 2 months, 25/26 with behavioural methods versus 6/13 with psychoeducation; ARR 0.5, RR 2.1, NNT 2 95% CI 2 to 5). We found one subsequent RCT which may be relevant.[48] It will be appraised for the next issue of *Clinical Evidence*.

Harms: None reported.

Comment: The first trial found low correlation between the different measures of compliance. The second trial also included some people with non-psychotic chronic psychiatric disorders and some people who were not taking antipsychotic medication. Both trials involved small numbers of people.

OPTION BEHAVIOURAL THERAPY

One RCT found that behavioural interventions improved adherence to antipsychotic medication compared with usual treatment. One RCT found that behavioural interventions improved adherence compared with psychoeducational therapy.

Benefits: We found no systematic review. **Versus usual treatment:** We found one RCT (36 men).[46] The behavioural training method comprised being told the importance of complying with antipsychotic medication and instructions on how to take medication. Each participant was given a self-monitoring spiral calendar, which featured a dated slip of paper for each dose of antipsychotic. Adherence was estimated by pill counts. After 3 months fewer people had high pill adherence after usual treatment compared with behaviour therapy (figures not presented). **Versus psychoeducational therapy:** see above.

Schizophrenia

Harms: None reported.

Comment: See above.

GLOSSARY

Compliance therapy A treatment based on cognitive behaviour therapy and motivational interviewing techniques with a view to improving concordance to medication.

Substantive changes since last issue of Clinical Evidence

Chlorpromazine Updated systematic review[7] includes three additional RCTs (total 45 RCTs); no change in conclusion.

Clozapine Updated systematic review[26] includes four additional RCTs (total 8 RCTs); no change in conclusion.

Continued treatment with antipsychotic drugs Three additional systematic reviews (total 8 systematic reviews); no change in conclusion.[9–33]

Additional RCTs have subsequently been identified and may be included in future issues of *Clinical Evidence*.

REFERENCES

1. Andreasen NC. Symptoms, signs and diagnosis of schizophrenia. *Lancet* 1995;346:477–481.
2. Cannon M, Jones P. Neuroepidemiology: schizophrenia. *J Neurol Neurosurg Psychiatry* 1996;61:604–613.
3. Jablensky A, Sartorius N, Ernberg G, et al. Schizophrenia: manifestations, incidence and course in different cultures. A World Health Organisation ten-country study. *Psychol Med* 1992;monograph supplement 20:1–97.
4. Hegarty JD, Baldessarini RJ, Tohen M, Waternaux C, Oepen G. One hundred years of schizophrenia: a meta-analysis of the outcome literature. *Am J Psychiatry* 1994;151:1409–1416.
5. Johnstone EC. Schizophrenia: problems in clinical practice. *Lancet* 1993; 341:536–538.
6. Thornley B, Adams C. Content and quality of 2000 controlled trials in schizophrenia over 50 years. *BMJ* 1998;317:1181–1184.
7. Thornley B, Adams CE, Awad G. Chlorpromazine versus placebo for those with schizophrenia. In: The Cochrane Library, Issue 2, 2000. Oxford: Update Software. Search date 1999; primary sources Biological Abstracts; Embase; Medline; Psyclit; SciSearch; Cochrane Library; Cochrane Schizophrenia Groups register; and hand searches of reference lists; and personal contact with pharmaceutical companies and authors of trials.
8. Quraishi S, David A. Depot haloperidol decanoate for schizophrenia. In: The Cochrane Library, Issue 2, 2000. Oxford: Update Software. Search date 1998; primary sources Biological Abstracts; Embase; Medline; Psyclit; SciSearch; Cochrane Library; reference lists; authors of studies; pharmaceutical companies.
9. Quraishi S, David A. Depot pipothiazine palmitate and undeclynate for schizophrenia. In: The Cochrane Library, Issue 2, 2000. Oxford: Update Software. Search strategy 1998; primary sources Biological Abstracts; Cochrane Library; Cochrane Schizophrenia Group's Register; Embase; Medline; and Psyclit; hand searches of reference lists; and personal communication with pharmaceutical companies.
10. Bagnall A-M, Fenton M, Lewis R, Leitner ML, Kleijnen J. Molindone for schizophrenia and severe mental illness. In: The Cochrane Library, Issue 2, 2000. Oxford: Update Software. Search date 1999; primary sources; Biological Abstracts; The Cochrane Library Central, The Cochrane Schizophrenia Group's Register, Cinahl; Embase; Psyclit; and pharmaceutical databases and hand searches of reference lists and personal contact with authors of trials.
11. Fenton M, Murphy B, Wood J, Bagnell A-M, Schou P, Leitner M. Loxapine for schizophrenia. In: The Cochrane Library, Issue 2, 2000. Oxford: Update Software. Search date 1999; primary sources Biological Abstracts; The Cochrane Library; The Cochrane Schizophrenia Group's Register; Embase; Lilacs; Psyndex; and PsycLIT; and hand searches of reference lists.
12. Sultana A, McMonagle T. Pimozide for schizophrenia or related psychoses. In: The Cochrane Library, Issue 2, 2000. Oxford: Update Software. Search date 1999; Biological Abstracts; The Cochrane Schizophrenia Group's Register; Embase; Janssen-Cilag UK's register of studies; Medline; and hand searches of reference lists and personal contact with pharmaceutical companies.
13. Joy CB, Mumby-Croft R, Joy LA. Polyunsaturated fatty acid (fish or evening primrose oil) for schizophrenia. In: The Cochrane Library, Issue 2, 2000. Oxford: Update Software. Search date 2000; primary sources Biological Abstracts; Cinahl; The Cochrane Library; The Cochrane Schizophrenia Group's Register; Embase; and Psyclit; and hand searches of reference lists; and personal contact with the authors.
14. Duggan L, Fenton M, Dardennes RM, El-Dosoky A, Indran S. Olanzapine for schizophrenia. In: The Cochrane Library, Issue 2, 2000. Oxford: Update Software. Search date June 1998; primary sources Biological Abstracts; Embase; Medline; Psyclit; Cochrane Library; and hand searches of reference lists and conference abstracts; personal communication with authors of trials and pharmaceutical companies.
15. Leucht S, Pitschel-Walx G, Abraham D, Kissling W. Efficacy and extrapyramidal side-effects of the new antipsychotics olanzapine, quetiapine, ripseridone and sertindole compared to conventional antipsychotics and placebo. A meta-analysis of randomised controlled trials. *Schizophr Res* 1999; 35:51–68. Search date 1999; primary sources Medline; Current Contents; and hand searches of reference lists; and personal communication with pharmaceutical companies.
16. Tuunainen A, Gilbody SM. Newer atypical antipsychotic medication versus clozapine for

schizophrenia. In: The Cochrane Library, Issue 2, 2000. Oxford: Update Software. Search date May 1998; primary sources Biological Abstracts; Cochrane Schizophrenia Group's register; Cochrane Library; Embase; Lilacs; Medline; Psyclit; and hand searches of reference lists; and personal contact with authors of trials and pharmaceutical companies.
17. Revicki D, Genduso L, Hamilton S, Ganoczy D, and Beasley C. Olanzapine versus haloperidol in the treatment of schizophrenia and other psychotic disorders: quality of life and clinical outcomes of a randomized clinical trial. *Qual Life Res* 1999;8: 417–426.
18. Srisurapanont M, Disayavanish C, Taimkaew K. Quetiapine for schizophrenia. In: The Cochrane Library, Issue 2, 2000. Oxford: Update Software. Search date 1998; primary sources Biological Abstracts; Embase; Medline; Psyclit; Cochrane Library; Cinahl; Sigle; Sociofile; hand searches of journals; personal communication with authors of studies and pharmaceutical companies.
19. Copolov DL, Link CGG, Kowalcyk B. A multicentre, double-blind, randomized comparison of quetiapine (ICI 204,636, "Seroquel") and haloperidol in schizophrenia. *Psychol Med* 2000; 30:95–105.
20. Barbui C. Quetiapine for schizophrenia. (Commentary). *Evid Based Mental Health* 1999;2: 52.
21. Kennedy E, Song F, Hunter R, Clarke Q, Gilbody S. Risperidone versus typical antipsychotic medication for schizophrenia. In: The Cochrane Library, Issue 2, 2000. Oxford: Update Software. Search date 1997; primary sources Biological Abstracts; The Cochrane Trials Register; Embase; Medline; and Psyclit; and hand searches of reference lists; and hand searches of reference lists; and personal communication with pharmaceutical companies.
22. Lopez Ibor JJ, Ayuso JL, Gutierrez M, et al. Risperidone in the treatment of chronic schizophrenia: multicenter study comparative to haloperidol. Actas Luso Esp Neurol Psiquiatr Cienc Afines 1996;24:165–172.
23. Bagnall A-M, Lewis RA, Leitner ML, Kleijnen J. Ziprasidone for schizophrenia and severe mental illness. In: The Cochrane Library, Issue 2, 2000. Oxford: Update Software. Search date 1999; primary sources Biological Abstracts; The Cochrane Library; The Cochrane Schizophrenia Group's Register; Embase; Lilacs; Psyndex; and Psyclit; pharmaceutical databases; and hand searches of reference lists; and personal contact with authors of trials.
24. Fenton M, Morris F, De Silva P, et al. Zotepine for schizophrenia. In: The Cochrane Library, Issue 2, 2000. Oxford: Update Software. Search date 1999; primary sources Biological Abstracts; The Cochrane Library; The Cochrane Schizophrenia Group's Register; Embase; Dialog Corporation Datastar service; Medline; and Psyclit; and hand searches of reference lists; and personal contact with authors of trials and pharmaceutical companies.
25. Wahlbeck K, Cheine M, Essali MA. Clozapine versus typical neuroleptic medication for schizophrenia. In: The Cochrane Library, Issue 2, 2000. Oxford: Update Software. Search date 1999; primary sources Biological Abstracts; Cochrane Schizophrenia Group's register; Cochrane Library; Embase; Lilacs; Medline; Psyclit; SciSearch — Science Citation Index; and hand searches of reference lists; and personal communication with pharmaceutical companies.
26. Tuunainen A, Gilbody SM. Newer atypical antipsychotic medication versus clozapine for schizophrenia. In: The Cochrane Library, Issue 2, 2000. Oxford: Update Software. Search date 1998; primary sources Biological Abstracts; Cochrane Schizophrenia Group's register; Cochrane Library; Embase; Lilacs; Medline; Psyclit; and hand searches of reference lists; and personal communicatio with authors of trials and pharmaceutical companies.
27. Honigfeld G, Arellano F, Sethi J, Bianchini A, Schein J. Reducing clozapine-related morbidity and mortality: five years experience of the Clozaril national registry. *J Clin Psychiatry* 1998;59(suppl 3):3–7.
28. Kumra S, Frazier JA, Jacobsen LK, et al. Childhood-onset schizophrenia. A double-blind clozapine-haloperidol comparison. *Arch Gen Psychiatry* 1996;53:1090–1097.
29. Gilbert PL, Harris MJ, McAdams LA, Jeste DV. Neuroleptic withdrawal in schizophrenic people: a review of the literature. *Arch Gen Psychiatry* 1995; 52:173–188. Search date not given; primary source Medline.
30. Adams CE, Eisenbruch M. Depot fluphenazine versus oral fluphenazine for those with schizophrenia. In: The Cochrane Library, Issue 2, 2000. Oxford: Update Software. Search date May 1995; primary sources Biological Abstracts; Cochrane Library; Cochrane Schizophrenia Group's register; Embase; Medline; Psyclit; Science Citation Index; hand searches of reference lists and personal communication with pharmaceutical companies.
31. Quraishi S, David A. Depot flupenthixol decanoate for schizophrenia or similar psychotic disorders. In: The Cochrane Library, Issue 2, 2000. Oxford: Update Software. Search date 1998; primary sources Biological Abstracts; Cochrane Library; Cochrane Schizophrenia Group's register; Embase; Medline; Psyclit; SciSearch; references, personal communication with authors of trials and pharmaceutical companies.
32. Quraishi S, David A. Depot fluspirilene for schizophrenia. In: The Cochrane Library, Issue 2, 2000. Oxford: Update Software. Search date 1998; primary sources Biological Abstracts; Cochrane Library; The Cochrane Schizophrenia Group's Register; Embase; Medline; and Psyclit; and hand searches of reference lists.
33. Quraishi S, David A. Depot perphenazine decanoate and enanthate for schizophrenia. In: The Cochrane Library, Issue 2, 2000. Oxford: Update Software. Search date 1998; primary sources Biological Abstracts; The Cochrane Library; The Cochrane Schizophrenia Group's Register; Embase; Medline; and Psyclit; and hand searches of reference lists; and personal communication with the pharmaceutical companies.
34. Coutinho E, Fenton M, Quraishi S. Zuclopenthixol decanoate for schizophrenia and other serious mental illnesses. In: The Cochrane Library, Issue 2, 2000. Oxford: Update software. Search date April 1998; primary sources Biological Abstracts 1982 to 1998, CINAHL 1982 to 1998), The Cochrane Library Issue 2, 2000, The Cochrane Schizophrenia Group's Register April 1998, Embase 1980 to 1998, Medline 1966 to 1998, Psyclit 1974 to 1998. References of all eligible studies were searched for further trials. The manufacturer of zuclopenthixol was contacted.
35. Jeste D, Gilbert P, McAdams L, Harris M. Considering neuroleptic maintenance and taper on a continuum: need for an individual rather than dogmatic approach. *Arch Gen Psychiatry* 1995; 52:209–212.
36. Pharaoh FM, Mari JJ, Streiner D. Family intervention for schizophrenia. In: The Cochrane

Library, Issue 2, 2000. Oxford: Update Software. Search date 1998; primary sources Medline; Embase; Cochrane Library; Cochrane Schizophrenia Group's Register of Trials; reference lists of articles.

37. McFarlane WR, Lukens E, Link B, et al. Multiple-family groups and psychoeducation in the treatment of schizophrenia. Arch Gen Psychiatry 1995;52:679–687.
38. Kemp R, Kirov G, Everitt B, Hayward P, David A. Randomised controlled trial of compliance therapy. 18-month follow-up. *Br J Psychiatry* 1998;172: 413–419.
39. Strang JS, Falloon IRH, Moss HB, Razani J, Boyd JL. Drug treatment and family intervention during the aftercare treatment of schizophrenics. *Psychopharmacology Bull* 1981;17:87–88.
40. Benton MK, Schroeder HE. Social skills training with schizophrenics: a meta-analytic evaluation. *J Consult Clin Psychol* 1990;58:741–747. Search date not given.
41. Corrigan PW. Social skills training in adult psychiatric populations: a meta-analysis. *J Behav Ther Exp Psychiatry* 1991;22:203–210. Search date 1988; primary sources Psychological Abstracts.
42. Jones C, Cormac I, Mota J, Campbell C. Cognitive behavioural therapy for schizophrenia. In: The Cochrane Library, Issue 2, 2000. Oxford: Update Software. Search date July 1998; primary sources Biological abstracts; Cochrane Schizophrenia Group's Register of Trials; Cinahl; Cochrane Library; Medline; Embase; Psyclit; Sigle; Sociofile; reference lists of articles; and personal communication with authors of trials.
43. Kemp R, Hayward P, Applewhaite G, Everitt B, David A. Compliance therapy in psychotic people: randomised controlled trial. *BMJ* 1996;312:345–349.
44. Xiong W, Phillips MR, Hu X, et al. Family-based intervention for schizophrenic people in China. A randomised controlled trial. *Br J Psychiatry* 1994; 165:239–247.
45. Zhang M, Wang M, Li J, Phillips MR. Randomised-control trial of family intervention for 78 first-episode male schizophrenic people. An 18-month study in Suzhou, Jiangsu. *Br J Psychiatry* 1994; 165:96–102.
46. Boczkowski JA, Zeichner A, DeSanto N. Neuroleptic compliance among chronic schizophrenic outpeople: an intervention outcome report. *J Consult Clin Psychol* 1985;53:666–671.
47. Azrin NH, Teichner G. Evaluation of an instructional program for improving medication compliance for chronically mentally ill outpatients. *Behaviour Res Ther* 1998;36:849–861.
48. Liberman RP, Wallace CJ, Blackwell G, Kopelowicz A, Vaccaro JV. et al. Mintz skills training versus psychological occupational therapy for persons with persistent schizophrenia. *Am J Psychiatry* 1998;155;8:1087–1091.

Stephen M Lawrie
Senior Clinical Research Fellow and
Honorary Consultant Psychiatrist
University of Edinburgh
Edinburgh
UK

Andrew McIntosh
Lecturer in Psychiatry
Department of Psychiatry
University of Edinburgh
Edinburgh
UK

Competing interests: Stephen Lawrie has been paid for speaking about critical appraisal, has had travel expenses for a conference reimbursed by Janssen the manufacturers of Risperidone, and has been paid for speaking about critical appraisal and chairing a symposium by Eli Lilly, the manufacturer of olanzapine.

TABLE 1 **Continued treatment with antipsychotic drugs: choice of drugs (see text, p 76).**

Review	Search Date	Number of RCTs	Comparisons	Main Conclusion
30	1995	6	Oral v depot fluphenazine	No significant difference
8	1998	7	Haloperidol decanoate *v* other depots	No significant difference
31	1998	8	Flupenthixol decanoate *v* other depots	No significant difference
9	1998	7	Pipothiazine palmitate *v* other depots	No significant difference
9	1998	2	Pipothiazine palmitate *v* oral antipsychotics	No significant difference
32	1998	1	Fluspirilene decanoate *v* oral chlorpromazine	No significant difference
32	1998	3	Fluspirilene decanoate *v* other depots	No significant difference
33	1998	1	Perphenazine enanthate *v* clopenthixol decanoate	No significant difference
12	1999	11	Pimozide *v* standard antipsychotics	No significant difference
14	1998	1	Olanzapine *v* standard antipsychotics	No significant difference
34	1998	3	Zuclopenthixol decanoate *v* other depots	People taking zuclopenthixol had lower relapse rates over 12 weeks to 1 year
25	1999	19	Clozapine *v* standard antipsychotics	Relapse rates up to 12 weeks were lower with clozapine

INDEX